2016 年度中医药国际合作专项
世界传统疗法研究与国际合作示范基地
资助出版

传统疗法实用技术手册

主　编　关雪峰　杨关林

·北京·

图书在版编目（CIP）数据

传统疗法实用技术手册 / 关雪峰，杨关林主编 .—
北京：人民卫生出版社，2023.4
ISBN 978-7-117-33492-1

Ⅰ.①传… Ⅱ.①关… ②杨… Ⅲ.①中医疗法 - 手
册 Ⅳ.①R242-62

中国版本图书馆 CIP 数据核字（2022）第 156338 号

人卫智网	www.ipmph.com	医学教育、学术、考试、健康，
		购书智慧智能综合服务平台
人卫官网	www.pmph.com	人卫官方资讯发布平台

传统疗法实用技术手册

Chuantong Liaofa Shiyong Jishu Shouce

主　　编：关雪峰　　杨关林
出版发行：人民卫生出版社（中继线 010-59780011）
地　　址：北京市朝阳区潘家园南里 19 号
邮　　编：100021
E - mail：pmph @ pmph.com
购书热线：010-59787592　010-59787584　010-65264830
印　　刷：北京铭成印刷有限公司
经　　销：新华书店
开　　本：710 × 1000　1/16　　印张：19
字　　数：331 千字
版　　次：2023 年 4 月第 1 版
印　　次：2023 年 5 月第 1 次印刷
标准书号：ISBN 978-7-117-33492-1
定价（含光盘）：82.00 元

Funded by
Special Project for International Cooperation in Traditional Chinese Medicine in 2016
Demonstration Base for International Cooperation and Research on World Traditional Therapies

Manual of Practical Technology for Traditional Therapy

Chief Editor: Guan Xuefeng   Yang Guanlin

PEOPLE'S MEDICAL PUBLISHING HOUSE
PMPH

《传统疗法实用技术手册》编委会

主　编　关雪峰　杨关林
副主编　吕　静　张　哲
编　委（按姓氏笔画排序）

王　洋　王　野　王欣欣　王晓彤　刘　创
刘文华　刘景峰　孙赫楠　李可大　李思琦
李福生　张　帆　张玉倩　郑海鹰　孟　健
胡晓丽　海　英　黄丽霞

序

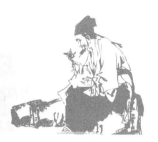

汉武文韬,张骞圣使,东起长安,马向西域,丝绸之路,此为缘起;

成于秦汉,南海为中,荣于唐宋,变于明清,海上丝绸,亦威且雄!

及兴废更迭,时至今日,一带一路,应运而生。夫岐黄仁术,华夏瑰宝,得天机而不敢自用,济天下而不吝交融,故借"一带一路"之东风,成本书之作,以广结青囊之友,普救含灵之苦,助力命运共同体之缔造。

余览此书,凡列四章,每章五节,每节一法。首章针法,并不列常见如毫针者,盖毫针可参之书,汗牛充栋,无新意耳!而遴选者,眼针、梅花针、火针、耳针、过梁针也,其眼针一法,首创于吾院彭老静山,疗效卓著,享誉海外。至于灸法、药浴、熥疗法各章节,亦搜罗百家,参阅各说,删繁正讹,散列者聚之,杂乱者理之,模棱者明之,稿凡数易,方成此书,实为辛苦有得之作,可启同道思考,以引真玉,可供海外共享,慧见东方。

"将升岱岳,非径奚为?欲诣扶桑,无舟莫适。"而欲达岐黄彼岸,欲天下皆认中医,所以依凭者,愚以为大抵有三:一曰志。个人之志乃修身立业之根,国家之志乃政策导向之本,志向明确,则行止有度,取舍相宜。二曰勇。凡医之大才,多与流俗相左,功成之前,栋梁与朽木实难辨也。而当事之人,应以万夫莫开之勇,忍不遇之屈,容嘲讽之辱,勇担当而能屈伸,知不足而自信,个人如此,国家亦如此,不因西学之风而怯懦畏惧,不因所趋者众而讨好倚靠,当立足疗效,积淀文化,继承创新,厚积薄发。三曰恒。为医者众,良医难得,非聪明不足,实用功未到也。当循序渐进,脚踏实地,精益求精;于中医走向世界而言,本土之士尚不得尽知其妙,尚不能尽信其功,期文化殊途者信之用之,难矣!当搭建平台,融合发展,启发交流,耐心推广。

冀本书早日付梓,以飨读者,亦待指正批评,勉之共进!

关雪峰

2022 年 1 月

Foreword

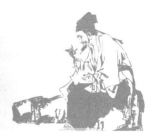

The Silk Road, from Chang'an (Xi'an now) to the west lands, was initiated by Emperor Wu in the Han Dynasty and started by Envoy Zhang Qian.

The great Maritime Silk Road, with the South China Sea as its center, was formed in the Qin and Han Dynasties, thrived in the Tang and Song Dynasties, and changed in the Ming and Qing Dynasties.

After vicissitudes, the Belt and Road Initiative comes into being nowadays. Traditional Chinese Medicine (TCM) is a great treasure for Chinese people. We are willing to share such a treasure with the world without reservation to save more people's lives. Therefore, with the opportunity of Belt and Road Initiative, I write this book to share it with all comrades and friends with the same ambition, to save people from sufferings, and to build a community of shared future for mankind.

This book is divided into four chapters, each of which has five sections, with one therapy discussed in each section. The first chapter of acupuncture does not list the common methods such as filiform needle method, because there are so many books about it and there is nothing new to be included in this book. While other methods of acupuncture are included such as periocular acupuncture, plum-blossom needle therapy, fire needle therapy, auricular acupuncture and penetration needle therapy. For example, the periocular acupuncture, created by Peng Jingshan in our hospital, is renowned overseas for its outstanding curative effects. As for chapters of moxibustion, medicated bath and Tong therapy, lots of schools and theories are included and referred to simplify the complex statements, to correct the wrong ones, to gather the scattered ones, to organize the tanglesome ones, and to clear the ambiguous ones. This book is the final version after several modifications, which can be used to inspire new and valuable thoughts and shared with the world to demonstrate the oriental wisdom.

"How can you go up high mountains without a path? How can you go to Fusang without a boat?" If you want to make achievements and want the world to recognize TCM, there are, I think, three crucial factors.First, it is ambition. As for individuals, ambition is the foundation of self-cultivation and career; as for a country, ambition is the basis of policies and guidelines.Only with clear ambition, will both individuals and countries behave with manners and make suitable choices.Second, it is bravery.The great talented doctors always hold different views from their peers.Before the great doctors become successful, it is difficult to distinguish them from the common ones.The great doctors are those with extraordinary bravery who can tolerate the frustration of not being recognized and respected, can take responsibilities bravely and make concession suitably, and can still keep self-confidence with knowledge of their own shortcomings.It is also true of a country.A country should not become timid or fearful for the prevalence of Western knowledge, and should not flatter or rely on Western knowledge for its popularity.A country should inherit and innovate its own medicine based on curative effects and continue to accumulate experience to thrive it some day.Third, it is perseverance.There are many doctors, but the good ones are rare.The reason is not that they are not intelligent enough, but that they do not make enough efforts.A good doctor should perfect their skills step by step in practice; as to the emergence of TCM to the world, it is definitely difficult for those of other culture to trust and use it if the native scholars do not fully understand and believe in the advantages and merits of the medicine! A platform should be established to integrate different development, to inspire communication, and to patiently promote it.

I hope that this book will be available for readers soon, and that any of you can correct possible errors in it for our mutual advance!

Guan Xuefeng
January 2022

前　言

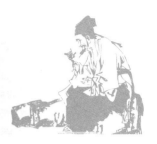

　　世界传统疗法是在人类文明历史长河中流传下来的珍贵财富,为现代医学的进步与发展奠定了基础。"精诚所至,金石为开",世界传统疗法的继承和规范化发展是我们不可推卸的责任。2016年世界传统疗法研究与国际合作示范基地搭建了3个世界传统疗法培训基地和3个世界传统疗法实训基地,创新了培训与实训相结合的远程教学模式。为进一步探索传统医学国际合作新模式,培养国际化复合型人才队伍,也为让更多人了解并受益于传统疗法,特编写《传统疗法实用技术手册》。

　　本书精心遴选针法、灸法、药浴、熥疗法四类20种传统疗法,在编写过程中注重科学性、实用性,既适合国内外中医院校学生、专业医务工作者培训学习,也适合世界传统医学爱好者学习使用。

　　针法和灸法是目前运用最多的两种传统疗法,常被并称为"针灸"。《史记》所载神医扁鹊起死回生,用针灸治好虢太子"尸厥"的故事,可谓家喻户晓。2010年,联合国教科文组织将"中医针灸"列入《人类非物质文化遗产代表作名录》。如今,针灸在全世界大放异彩,据国务院新闻办公室2018年10月发表的《中国的中医针灸》统计,中医针灸已传播到183个国家和地区,从业人员已达到38万。据世界卫生组织统计,29个国家已设立了世界传统医学的法律法规,针灸已进入国际医疗体系。

　　药浴有着鲜明的地域特点,在很长一段时间里并没有广泛流传,但我们必须承认药浴在保障民众的生命健康和防治疾病方面发挥了重要作用。联合国教科文组织保护非物质文化遗产政府间委员会第十三届常会于2018年11月26日至12月1日在毛里求斯首都路易港召开,通过决议,将中国申报的"藏医药浴法——中国藏族有关生命健康和疾病防治的知识与实践"列入联合国教科文组织《人类非物质文化遗产代表作名录》,证明了药浴是世界传统疗法不可或缺的一部分,本书介绍了包括藏药浴在内的5种疗法,希望可以推广药浴走向世界。

熥疗法是传统医学遗产中重要的一部分,它具有疗效高、副作用小和治疗方便等优点,不仅适宜于医院,而且适宜于广大人民群众在家庭中进行自我治疗,是使用较为广泛的一种传统疗法。

本书介绍的 20 种疗法是传统疗法中最具代表性的,并不能囊括所有疗法,还有更多的方法亟待我们去发掘、继承。希望本书可以在促进世界传统疗法文化的传播,提升中医药的国际影响力和社会认可度,以及规范治疗手法,提升医生的专业水平、群众的辨别能力,消除某些对于传统疗法的误解等方面作出贡献。限于水平及能力,有误之处敬请读者批评指正!

编委会

2022 年 1 月

Preface

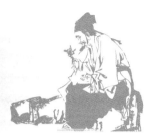

World traditional therapies are valuable assets handed down in the long history of human civilization, which has laid a foundation for the progress and development of modern medicine.Faith will move mountains, and it is our unshirkable responsibility to promote the inheritance and standardized development of world traditional therapies.In 2016, Demonstration Base for International Cooperation and Research on World Traditional Therapies set up three world traditional therapy training bases and three world traditional therapy practical bases, which innovated the distance learning model combining training and practice.In order to further explore the new mode of international cooperation in traditional medicine, cultivate an international team of inter-disciplinary talents and let more people know and benefit from traditional therapies, the *Manual of Practical Technology for Traditional Therapy* is specially compiled.

This book introduces 20 kinds of traditional therapies under 4 categories containing acupuncture, moxibustion, medicated bath and Tong therapy.During the writing process, we put the emphasis on scientificity and practicality of the contents.Therefore, this book can be used for the training of the students from TCM colleges and universities and medical professionals at home and abroad, and can also meet the learning needs of the world traditional medicine lovers.

Now, the acupuncture therapy and the moxibustion therapy are the two most commonly-used traditional therapies, which can be together called "Acupuncture and Moxibustion".The story of the highly-skilled doctor Bian Que who treated corpse-like syncope disease of prince of the Guo state by the Acupuncture and Moxibustion described in the *Records of the Grand Historian* is well known.In 2010, United Nations Educational Scientific and Cultural Organization(UNESCO) has added "Acupuncture and moxibustion of traditional Chinese medicine" to its *Representative List of The Intangible Cultural Heritage of Humanity*.Now, the acupuncture and moxibustion is gaining popularity all over the world.According to the statistics of the *Acupuncture and Moxibustion of Traditional Chinese Medicine in China* published by the Information Office of the State Council in October 2018, acupuncture and moxibustion of traditional Chinese medicine has spread to 183 countries and regions with 380,000 practitioners.According to the statistics of the World Health Organization, 29 countries have established laws and regulations on world traditional medicine, and the acupuncture and moxibustion has entered the international medical system.

The medicated bath has distinct regional characteristics, and is not widely spread over a long period of time.However, it must be admitted that the medicated bath plays an important role in protecting public life and health and preventing and treating diseases.The 13th regular meeting of UNESCO Intergovernmental Committee for the Safeguarding of the Intangible Cultural Heritage was held between November 26, 2018 and December 1, 2018 in the capital of Mauritius, Port Louis, and passed a resolution to add "Lum medicinal bathing of Sowa Rigpa, knowledge and practices concerning life, health and illness prevention and treatment among the Tibetan people in China" declared by China to UNESCO *Representative List of The Intangible Cultural Heritage of Humanity*, proving that the medicated bath is an integral part of the world traditional therapies.This book introduces 5 kinds of therapies including Tibetan medicated bath therapy, and we hope to promote the medicated bath to the world.

Tong therapy is an important part of the traditional medical heritage, and has many advantages such as rapid effect, small side effect and convenient treatment. The therapy not only can be used in hospital, but also in the family for self-treatment, which is a relatively widely-used traditional therapy.

The 20 therapies described in this book are the most representative traditional therapies.Not all traditional therapies are described here, and there are many methods that need to be discovered and inherited.It is hoped that this book can contribute to promoting the spread of world traditional therapies, enhancing the international influence and social recognition of TCM, standardizing treatment techniques, improving the professional level of doctors and the discrimination ability of the public, and eliminating some misunderstandings about traditional therapies.Due to limited academic level and professional capacity, omissions are unavoidable.So criticisms are welcomed from readers!

Editorial Board

January 2022

目　　录
Table of Contents

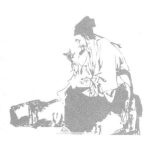

15

第一章 针 法
Chapter 1 Acupuncture

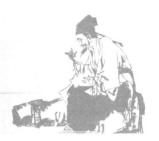

第一节 眼 针
Section 1 Periocular Acupuncture

眼针疗法是辽宁中医药大学附属医院彭静山教授首创的一种微针疗法。

Periocular acupuncture is a micro-needle therapy initiated by Professor Peng Jingshan from the Affiliated Hospital of Liaoning University of Traditional Chinese Medicine.

眼针疗法是在眼眶内外特定的穴区进行针刺等刺激，以治疗全身疾病的一种方法。

Periocular acupuncture is a method for treating whole body's disease by means of stimulating specific acupoint area inside and outside the orbit of eyes through needling.

治疗时按照脏腑辨证、经络辨证、三焦辨证及观眼识证4种取穴原则进行取穴。

During the treatment, the following four acupoint selection principles should be based on:syndrome differentiation of zang-fu organs, syndrome differentiation of meridians and collaterals, syndrome differentiation of sanjiao theory, and syndrome differentiation based on examining eyes.

一、眼针的分区定穴(图 1-1)

I. Area Division and Acupoint Location for Periocular Acupuncture (Fig. 1-1)

(一) 分区
(I) Area Division

双眼平视正前方,以瞳孔为中心做水平线及垂线,即从瞳孔发出的上、下、

1

内、外 4 条线将眼球等分为 4 个区域,再从该 4 个区域各引一条平分线,此时以瞳孔为中心的 8 条线将眼球等分为 8 个区域,该 8 条线称为分区定位线。

First, make a horizontal line and a vertical line in the center of pupil with eyes looking at front horizontally, such that eyeball is divided into four areas by four lines, i.e., up, down, inside and outside given out from pupil. Then cite a bisector for each area, such that the eyeball is divided into eight areas in the center of pupil. The eight lines are called partition positioning lines.

内上方的平分线为分区定位 1 线。

The bisector in the medial superior quadrant of eyeball is partition positioning line 1.

瞳孔正上方的垂线为分区定位 2 线。

The vertical line just above pupil is partition positioning line 2.

外上方的平分线为分区定位 3 线。

The bisector in the lateral superior quadrant of eyeball is partition positioning line 3.

瞳孔至目外眦的水平线为分区定位 4 线。

The horizontal line from pupil to outer canthus is partition positioning line 4.

外下方的平分线为分区定位 5 线。

Tthe bisector in the lateral inferior quadrant of eyeball is partition positioning line 5.

瞳孔正下方的垂线为分区定位 6 线。

The vertical line just below pupil is partition positioning line 6.

内下方的平分线为分区定位 7 线。

The bisector in the medial inferior quadrant of eyeball is partition positioning line 7.

瞳孔至目内眦的水平线为分区定位 8 线。

The horizontal line from pupil to medial canthus is partition positioning line 8.

再以瞳孔为中心发出 8 条平分线,将上述 8 个区域等分为 16 个小区域。

At last, divide the above-mentioned 8 areas into 16 areas by the 8 bisectors giving out in the center of pupil.

分区时,以分区定位 1 线为中心,将其邻近的 2 个小区域划分为 1 区;以分区定位 2 线为中心,将其邻近的 2 个小区域划分为 2 区。

When dividing areas, partition positioning line 1 is taken as the center to combine 2 small adjacent areas to form Area 1; partition positioning line 2 is taken as the center to combine 2 small adjacent areas to form Area 2.

同理,陆续可以划分 3 区 ~8 区。

Similarly, Areas 3-8 can form in succession.

(二) 定穴
(Ⅱ) Acupoint Location

沿自 1 区至 8 区的方向,划分如下:

Along the direction from Area 1 to Area 8, the visceral acupoint areas can be located as the following:

1 区为肺大肠区。

Area 1 for lung and large intestine.

2 区为肾膀胱区。

Area 2 for kidney and bladder.

3 区为上焦区。

Area 3 for upper jiao.

4 区为肝胆区。

Area 4 for liver and gallbladder.

5 区为中焦区。

Area 5 for middle jiao.

6 区为心小肠区。

Area 6 for heart and small intestine.

7 区为脾胃区。

Area 7 for spleen and stomach.

8 区为下焦区。

Area 8 for lower jiao.

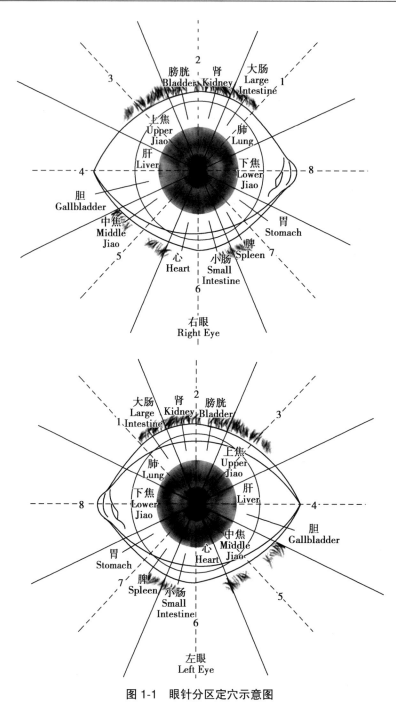

图 1-1 眼针分区定穴示意图

Fig. 1-1 Schematic diagram of periocular acupuncture partition positioning

二、操作技术

Ⅱ. Operation Techniques

(一) 操作前准备

(Ⅰ) Preparation Before Operation

1. 针具选择 宜用 29~33 号（0.26~0.34mm），0.5~1 寸（15~25mm）的一次性毫针。

1. Needling Instrument Selection Disposable filiform needles for acupuncture from No.29-33（0.26-0.34mm）and 0.5-1 cun（a Chinese unit of length equals 1/3 decimeter）（15-25mm）.

所选择的毫针针身应光滑、无锈蚀，针尖应锐利、无倒钩。

The body of the filiform needles selected should be smooth with no rusting. The needle point should be sharp with no barb.

2. 部位选择 在眼眶内外，选取穴区进行操作。

2. Position Selection Select acupoint area inside and outside the orbit of eye.

3. 体位选择 选择患者舒适，医者便于操作的治疗体位。

3. Posture Selection Select a treatment position which is comfortable for patient and is easy for doctor to operate.

4. 环境要求 环境应清洁卫生，避免污染。

4. Environment Requirements The environment should keep clean and hygienic with no contamination.

5. 消毒

5. Sterilization

（1）针具消毒：应选择高压蒸汽消毒法。

（1）Needle Sterilization：High pressure steam sterilization should be selected.

（2）部位消毒：应用含 75% 医用乙醇或 0.5%~1% 碘伏的棉签或棉球在施术部位消毒。

（2）Position Sterilization：The cotton swab or cotton ball with 75% medical ethanol or 0.5%-1% iodophor should be used to sterilize the operated sites.

（3）医者消毒：医者双手可先用肥皂水清洗干净，再用含 75% 医用乙醇或 0.5%~1% 碘伏的棉球擦拭。

（3）Sterilization of Doctor：The doctor should wash hands with soap and water firstly，then brush hands with cotton balls of 75% medical ethanol or 0.5%-1% iodophor to sterilize.

（二）施术方法

（Ⅱ）Application Methods

1. 眶内直刺法　以押手固定眼球，持针在紧贴眼眶内缘的穴区，垂直进针 0.5 寸（15mm）。

1. Straight Acupuncture inside Orbit　Use the hands to press and fix the eyeball. Hold needle in acupoint area which is near inner rim of the orbit，and insert vertically with 0.5 cun（15mm）.

2. 眶外平刺法　持针在距眼眶内缘 2mm 的穴区部位，进行平刺操作，刺入真皮，达至皮下组织，进针 0.5 寸（15mm），保持针体处于该穴区内。

2. Horizontal Acupuncture outside Orbit　Hold needle in the acupoint area where is 2mm far away from inner rim of the orbit，conduct horizontal insertion，and penetrate into derma，reach subcutaneous tissue. The depth of needling is about 0.5 cun（15mm），with the needle being kept in the acupoint area.

3. 点刺法　以押手固定眼睑，使之绷紧，持针在眼睑部选取穴区轻轻点刺 5~7 次，以不出血为度。

3. Pricking Acupuncture　Use the hands to press and fix the eyelid，so as to make it tight. Use needle to prick slightly at the selected acupoint area in the eyelid 5-7 times with no bleeding.

4. 双刺法　不论采取眶内直刺法或眶外平刺法，当刺入一针后，在其所处的穴区内，紧贴着针体旁，按同一方向，再刺入一针，均进针 0.5 寸（15mm）。

4. Double Acupuncture　For either of straight acupuncture inside the orbit or horizontal acupuncture outside the orbit，after inserting one needle，insert another one near the body of the needle at the same direction in the same acupoint area. Both should insert 0.5 cun（15mm）deep.

5. 眶内外合刺法　于同一穴区内，在眶内、眶外各刺一针，均进针 0.5 寸（15mm）。

5. Combined Acupuncture inside and outside Orbit　In the same acupoint area, at both the inside and outside of the orbit, one needle is taken to puncture 0.5 cun(15mm)deep.

6. 压穴法　于所选取的穴区内,使用点穴棒、三棱针柄等,按压眼眶内缘,以局部产生酸、麻、胀感为度,持续按压 15~30 分钟。

6. Pressing Acupoint　Press inner rim of eye 15-30 minutes continuously in the selected acupoint area by using an acupoint bar, or the handle of a three-edged needle. The intensity of operation should reach a point that the patient gets a sensation of local soreness, numbness and distension.

(三) 施术后处理

(Ⅲ) Treatment after Application

1. 行针技术要求　一般情况下,进针后不需行针;如果进针后针感不明显,可施以刮柄法或将针体提出 1/3,稍改变方向后再行刺入。

1. Technical Requirements for Manipulating Needles　Normally, after inserting needles, it's unnecessary to do any manipulations; if the needling sensation is not obvious after inserting needles, perform the technique of scraping the needle handle or change the direction slightly and then penetrate the needle again by taking one thirds of the needle body out.

2. 留针技术要求

2. Technical Requirements for Retaining Needles

(1) 静置留针法:留针期间不施行任何针刺手法,让针体留置在穴区内。

(1) Static Needle Retaining Method:In the period of retaining needle, don't do any manipulations, just let the needle body in the acupoint area.

一般情况下,留针时间宜在 15~60 分钟。

Normally, the needles should be retained for 15-60 minutes.

(2) 刮柄刺激法:留针期间内,如果局部得气感不明显,则可间歇重复施行刮柄法,以加强刺激。

(2) Handle-scraping Stimulation:During the retention period, if regional sensation of arrival of qi is not obvious, this method can be repeated at interval to enhance stimulation.

一般情况下，在 15~30 分钟内，宜间歇行针 1~2 次，每次 0.5~1 分钟。

Normally, within 15-30 minutes, it is suitable to manipulate the needle 1-2 times, 0.5-1 minutes each time.

3. 出针技术要求　以刺手的拇、示二指捏持针柄，轻轻转动后缓慢出针 1/2，然后慢慢拔出，拔针后即刻用干棉球按压针孔，宜按压 1~3 分钟。

3. Technical Requirements for Drawing out Needles　Use thumb and index finger to hold the handle of needle, draw one half of needle out after gently rotating and then draw the rest out slowly. After drawing all the needle out, use cotton ball to press the acupuncture hole immediately, perfectly 1-3 minutes.

4. 眼针治疗间隔及疗程　眼针技术治疗时，宜每日 1 次，连续治疗 10~14 天为 1 个疗程，休息 2 天后，可进行下一疗程。

4. Interval and Course of Treatment of Periocular Acupuncture　Periocular acupuncture treatment should be done once a day and 10-14 days treatment in succession makes a course of treatment. After two-day rest, next course can be carried out.

三、临床应用

Ⅲ. Clinical Application

（一）适应范围
（Ⅰ）Application Range

1. 内科　中风、头痛、眩晕、面瘫、失眠、高血压、三叉神经痛、膈肌痉挛、血管性痴呆、抑郁症、癫痫、重症肌无力、眼肌麻痹、不宁腿综合征、吉兰 - 巴雷综合征、支气管哮喘、面肌痉挛、胆囊炎、溃疡性结肠炎、急性胃肠炎、胆道蛔虫病等。

1. In Internal Medicine　Apoplexy, headache, vertigo, facial paralysis, insomnia, hypertension, trigeminal neuralgia, diaphragmatic spasm, vascular dementia, depressive disorder, epilepsy, myasthenia gravis, ophthalmoplegia, restless leg syndrome, Guillain-Barré syndrome, bronchial asthma, facial spasm, cholecystitis, ulcerative colitis, acute gastroenteritis, biliary ascariasis, etc.

2. 骨伤科　颈椎病、肩周炎、腰椎间盘突出症、坐骨神经痛、落枕、急性腰扭伤等。

2. In Osteology and Traumatology　Cervical spondylosis, scapulohumeral periarthritis, prolapse of lumber intervertebral disc, sciatica, stiff neck, acute lumbar muscle sprain, etc.

3. 妇科 痛经、月经不调等。

3. In Gynecology Dysmenorrhea, menstrual disorders, etc.

4. 儿科 疳积、小儿腹泻、百日咳等。

4. In Pediatric Infantile malnutrition, infantile diarrhea, whooping cough, etc.

5. 皮肤科 黄褐斑、蝴蝶斑、痤疮、带状疱疹等。

5. In Dermatology Chloasma, butterfly rash, acne, herpes zoster, etc.

6. 外科 肾结石、胆结石、血栓闭塞性脉管炎等。

6. In Surgery Renal calculus, gallstone, thromboangiitis obliterans, etc.

7. 五官科 突发性耳聋、中心性视网膜炎、近视、眼肌麻痹、弱视等。

7. In Ophthalmology and Otorhinolaryngology Sudden deafness, central serous chorioretinopathy, near sight, ophthalmoplegia, amblyopia, etc.

（二）处方示例

（Ⅱ）Prescription Samples

1. 中风

1. Apoplexy

（1）中经络

（1）Apoplexy Involving Meridians and Collaterals

1）风痰阻络证

1）Wind-phlegm Obstructing Collaterals

主穴：上焦区、下焦区。

Major Acupoints: Upper jiao area, lower jiao area.

配穴：脾区、肝区。

Supplement Acupoints: Spleen area, liver area.

2）肝阳暴亢证

2）Hyperactivity of Liver Yang

主穴：上焦区、下焦区。

Major Acupoints: Upper jiao area, lower jiao area.

配穴:肝区、肾区。

Supplement Acupoints: Liver area, kidney area.

3）痰热腑实证

3）Syndrome of Excessive Fu-Viscera Caused by Phlegm-Heat

主穴:上焦区、下焦区。

Major Acupoints: Upper jiao area, lower jiao area.

配穴:脾区、大肠区。

Supplement Acupoints: Spleen area, large intestine area.

4）气虚血瘀证

4）Syndrome of Blood Stasis Due to Qi Deficiency

主穴:上焦区、下焦区。

Major Acupoints: Upper jiao area, lower jiao area.

配穴:心区、脾区。

Supplement Acupoints: Heart area, spleen area.

5）阴虚风动证

5）Syndrome of Wind Stirring Due to Yin Deficiency

主穴:上焦区、下焦区。

Major Acupoints: Upper jiao area, lower jiao area.

配穴:肝区、肾区。

Supplement Acupoints: Liver area, kidney area.

（2）中脏腑

（2）Apoplexy Involving Zang-Fu Organs

1）风火闭窍证

1）Syndrome of Wind-Fire Blocking Orifices

主穴:上焦区、下焦区。

Major Acupoints: Upper jiao area, lower jiao area.

配穴：心区、肝区。

Supplement Acupoints：Heart area，liver area.

2）痰火闭窍证

2）Syndrome of Phlegm-Fire Blocking Orifices

主穴：上焦区、下焦区。

Major Acupoints：Upper jiao area，lower jiao area.

配穴：心区、脾区。

Supplement Acupoints：Heart area，spleen area.

3）痰湿蒙窍证

3）Apoplexy with Syndrome of Phlegm-Damp Clouding Orifices

主穴：上焦区、下焦区。

Major Acupoints：Upper jiao area，lower jiao area.

配穴：脾区、肝区。

Supplement Acupoints：Spleen area，liver area.

4）元气衰败证

4）Syndrome of Primordial Qi Decline

主穴：上焦区、下焦区。

Major Acupoints：Upper jiao area，lower jiao area.

配穴：肾区、心区、脾区。

Supplement Acupoints：Kidney area，heart area，spleen area.

2. 眩晕

2. Vertigo

（1）肝阳上亢证

（1）Syndrome of Upper Hyperactivity of Liver Yang

主穴：上焦区。

Major Acupoints：Upper jiao area.

配穴：肝区、肾区。

Supplement Acupoints:Liver area,kidney area.

（2）痰浊中阻证

（2）Syndrome of Phlegm-Turbidity Obstructing Middle Jiao

主穴:上焦区。

Major Acupoints:Upper jiao area.

配穴:肝区、脾区。

Supplement Acupoints:Liver area,spleen area.

（3）气血亏虚证

（3）Syndrome of Deficiency of Both Qi and Blood

主穴:上焦区。

Major Acupoints:Upper jiao area.

配穴:脾区、胃区。

Supplement Acupoints:Spleen area,stomach area.

（4）肾精不足证

（4）Syndrome of Insufficiency of Kidney Essence

主穴:上焦区。

Major Acupoints:Upper jiao area.

配穴:肾区、下焦区。

Supplement Acupoints:Kidney area,lower jiao area.

3. 面瘫

3. Facial Paralysis

（1）风寒袭络证

（1）Syndrome of Collateral Invaded by Wind-Cold

主穴:上焦区。

Major Acupoints:Upper jiao area.

配穴:肺区。

Supplement Acupoints:Lung area.

（2）风热袭络证

(2) Syndrome of Collateral Invaded by Wind-heat

主穴：上焦区。

Major Acupoints：Upper jiao area.

配穴：肺区。

Supplement Acupoints：Lung area.

（3）风痰阻络证

(3) Syndrome of Collateral Obstructed by Wind-phlegm

主穴：上焦区。

Major Acupoints：Upper jiao area.

配穴：脾区。

Supplement Acupoints：Spleen area.

（4）气虚血瘀证

(4) Syndrome of Blood Stasis Due to Qi Deficiency

主穴：上焦区。

Major Acupoints：Upper jiao area.

配穴：脾区。

Supplement Acupoints：Spleen area.

（5）肝胆湿热证

(5) Syndrome of Dampness-Heat of Liver and Gallbladder

主穴：上焦区。

Major Acupoints：Upper jiao area.

配穴：肝区、胆区。

Supplement Acupoints：Liver area, gallbladder area.

（三）禁忌证

(Ⅲ) Contraindications

1.眼区有破损感染者禁用。

1. Patient whose eye area is damaged or infected is prohibited to take this

therapy.

2. 精神病患者禁用。

2. Patient with psychosis is prohibited to take this therapy.

3. 传染病患者禁用。

3. Patient with infectious diseases is prohibited to take this therapy.

4. 金属过敏者禁用。

4. Patient allergic to metal is prohibited to take this therapy.

（四）注意事项

（Ⅳ）Precautions

1. 针刺注意事项

1. Precautions in Acupuncture

（1）注意防止发生晕针或晕血。

（1）Pay attention to fainting during acupuncture or blood phobia.

（2）注意防止发生局部出血或血肿。

（2）Pay attention to regional bleeding or hematoma.

（3）注意防止进针时伤及眼球。

（3）Pay attention to the eye injury when inserting the needle.

（4）点刺操作时，进针宜浅，手法宜轻、宜快。

（4）When doing the pricking acupuncture, the insertion of needle should be shallow and the manipulation should be light and fast.

（5）注意防止操作部位感染。

（5）Pay attention to infection of the operated position.

（6）孕妇及新产后慎用眼针疗法。

（6）Pregnant women and new mothers should use periocular acupuncture therapy cautiously.

（7）患者精神紧张、大汗后、劳累后或饥饿时慎用本疗法。

（7）Patients who are nervous, sweating, tired or hungry should use this therapy cautiously.

（8）震颤不止，躁动不安，眼睑肥厚者慎用。

（8）Patients with tremor, restlessness, eyelid hypertrophy should use this therapy cautiously.

2. 留针的注意事项
2. Precautions in Retaining Needles

（1）留针要因人而异。体弱者留针时间较短，体壮者可适当延长留针时间。

（1）The time of retaining needle should differ from man to man. For weak patients, the time should be short, and for strong patients, the time may be appropriately extended.

婴幼儿和躁动患者，以及其他难于合作者，不宜留针。

Infants and restlessness patients and patients who are not easy to cooperate are unsuitable to retain needle.

（2）留针要因时而异。夏季天气炎热，不宜久留针；冬季气候寒冷，适宜久留针。

（2）The time of retaining needle should differ from season to season. When the weather is hot in summer, the time should be shorter; when the weather is cold in winter, the time should be longer.

（3）留针要因病而异。病情轻、症状轻或经治疗症状已消失者，可以不留针或短时间留针。

（3）The time of retaining needle should be based on the condition of disease. Patients who have mild illness and symptoms or disappeared symptoms after treatment, don't need to retain the needle or it can be a short time.

病情重、症状顽固者宜久留针。

Patients who have serious illness or intractable symptoms can retain the needle for a longer time.

（4）留针要注意安全。留针期间要叮嘱患者及家属不要碰触留置在眼眶内外的毫针，以免折针、弯针。

（4）Pay attention to the safety when retaining needle. In the period of retention, urge patients and their families not to touch the filiform needle, so as not to break and bend needle.

对需要长期留针而又有严重心脑血管疾病者，须加强监护，以免发生意外。

Patients who need a long-term retention of needle and also have severe cardiovascular and cerebrovascular diseases should be given an intensive monitoring, so as to avoid accident.

（五）意外的处理方法

（Ⅴ）Treatment of Accidents

1. 晕针的处理　如有晕针发生，应立即停止针刺，将针全部起出，让患者平卧休息，并给予温开水或糖水，严重者予以吸氧、补液等急救措施。

1. Treatment of Fainting During Acupuncture　If fainting during acupuncture occurs, doctor should stop acupuncture immediately, pull all the needles out, let the patient lie on the back, have a rest and give him or her warm boiled water or sugar water. Give patient who has serious fainting the first aid measures such as oxygen inhalation and transfusion.

2. 出血的处理　眼周血管丰富，容易出血，出针时应注意按压针孔，如出现严重血肿，应先冷敷止血，再做热敷或揉按局部以促进瘀血吸收。

2. Treatment of Bleeding　Pay attention to press the acupuncture hole when drawing out needle because bleeding may occur due to a plenty of vessels around the eye. If severe hematoma occurs, cold compress should be done firstly to stop bleeding, then do hot compress or do regional rubbing in order to promote the absorption of blood stasis.

3. 弯针的处理　发现弯针后，不可再行提插、捻转等手法。

3. Treatment of Needle Bending　When the needle is bent, don't do manipulations such as lifting, inserting and twirling, etc.

应顺势慢慢退出。切忌强行拔针，以免将针断入体内。

The needle should be pulled out slowly. Don't pull the needle out forcibly, so as to avoid the needle broken into the position.

第二节　梅　花　针

Section 2　Plum-Blossom Needle

梅花针疗法，古称"毛刺""扬刺""浮刺""半刺"，将5~7枚6号或7号不锈钢针,依法捆扎在一根富有弹性的筷子(或小竹棒、小木棒等)一端(钻一小孔)的小孔内,露出针尖,捆成一束,像梅花的形状,或使用软柄、硬柄梅花针,术者右手握住针柄,在人体皮肤(应刺部位)上,运用一定的手法,只叩击皮肤,不伤及肌肉,以达到疏通经络、调节脏腑、祛邪扶正、防治疾病的一种外治疗法。

Plum-blossom needle therapy,being called as "skin needling", "quintuple needling", "superficial needling" or "half-needling" in ancient time,is an external therapy,in which,according to the convention,five to seven 6# or 7# stainless steel needles are bundled in a drilled hole at one end of a flexible chopstick(or a bamboo stick or a wooden stick,etc.),several sticks are bundled in a shape of plum blossom,with the needle tips pointing out. The handle of plum-blossom needle can be soft or hard. When practicing,the doctor holds the handle in his right hand and taps the patient on the skin in an area which needs operation but the muscles should not be hurt. The therapy can dredge meridians and collaterals, regulate functions of zang-fu organs,eliminate pathogenic factors,reinforce body resistance and prevent disease.

由于针数不同,故又有五星针(5枚)、七星针(7枚)之称。

According to the number of needles,it is called five-star needle(five needles) or seven-star needle(seven needles).

又因叩打在皮肤上,故又被人称为"皮刺针""皮肤针""丛针"。

The therapy is also called "skin puncture", "skin needling" or "bundled needling" because it taps on the skin.

一、梅花针刺激部位

Ⅰ. Stimulating Parts of Plum-Blossom Needle

梅花针可以刺激的部位有很多,除特定刺激部位外,还可根据中医经络学说选用经穴、阿是穴,随证选用刺激部位经穴,均可取得一定的疗效。

There are many parts on the human body that could be tapped and stimulated for plum-blossom needle. Apart from specific stimulating parts,we can choose the meridian points and Ashi points according to syndrome differentiated based on the TCM theory of meridians and collaterals,and the treatment effects can be also certain.

（一）梅花针刺激部位检查方法

（Ⅰ）Method to Choose Stimulating Parts of Plum-Blossom Needle

梅花针应用于临床治疗,其检查方法中脊柱两侧检查诊断法最具特色,即医师运用两手触按脊柱两侧,检查有无异常反应,如有条索状、结节状物或疱状软性物,可称为阳性反应检查或阳性物,即适宜用梅花针治疗。

When the plum-blossom needle is applied to clinical treatment, among its examining methods, a diagnostic method to examine both sides of the spinal column is unique. The doctor uses his or her hands to press both sides of the spinal column to check whether there is any abnormal reaction, such as soft cord-like, node-like or blister-like indicator, which can be taken as positive reactions or positive indicator, being suitable for treatment by plum-blossom needle.

这种异常反应在治疗中占有很重要的地位,检查发现的异常部位,即是治疗过程中的重点刺激部位。

Such abnormal reactions play an important role during the treatment, and the abnormal positions discovered through examining are the key stimulating parts in treatment.

在进行检查时,嘱患者露出整个背部和臀部,采取俯伏坐位,俯伏在检查台上,头向下低,背成弓形。

In examination, the doctor should ask the patient to take a prone position in an examining bed with the head bowed and the back arched, exposing the whole back and buttocks.

并嘱患者不可过于紧张,要全身放松,积极配合,否则会影响检查的结果,施术者应坐或站在患者的右后方。

During the examination, the patient should not be too nervous, with the body being relaxing, and coordinate with the doctor actively. Otherwise, the result of examination will be affected. The operator should sit or stand in the right rear of the patient.

检查方法归纳为叩、摸、推、压、捏五法。

Checking techniques are generalized into five methods, i.e. percussing, touching, pushing, pressing and pinching.

叩诊:又称"敲诊",即检查者将右手或左手示指、中指、环指、小指四个手指并拢,稍弯曲,如同西医叩诊一样,用适当的腕力,从上(颈椎开始)往下(至腰骶部为止)叩打,如果身体某部位有病,往往在叩诊时会在颈、胸、腰、骶部发现异常音响。

Percussing: It is also called "knocking". First, the examiner joins his or her index finger, middle finger, ring finger and little finger of right or left hand together and bends them slightly. And then, as the percussion in Western medicine, the examiner appropriately uses the wrist strength to knock the patient's body from top (cervical vertebra) to bottom (lumbosacral portion). If a certain position of the body is ill, there will be abnormal sounds detectable from the neck, chest, waist or sacrum during percussion.

摸诊:检查者以右手或左手摸患者的皮肤,主要是检查患者皮肤的温度、光洁度(粗糙)及湿润度等是否有异常。

Touching: The examiner touches the skin of the patient with his right or left hand to examine whether there is an abnormality in skin temperature, smoothness (toughness) and moisture.

推诊:检查者以右手或左手拇指压在患者脊柱两旁的一侧,用适当的压力,从下向上推。此法不但有助于诊断,而且有重要的治疗作用。

Pushing: The examiner presses one side of the patient's spinal column with his or her right or left hand and push up from bottom with adequate force. This method not only helps to make diagnosis but also has important therapeutic effect.

压诊:检查者右手或左手拇指在患者脊柱两侧及其他部位,用适当的压力按之。

Pressing: The examiner presses both sides of the patient's spinal column or other positions using the thumb of his or her right or left hand with adequate force.

在压诊时,如发现异常现象,则说明疾病的存在,并可预知疾病的预后及其进展情况。

Any abnormal phenomenon detected during pressing means that there is a disease and the prognosis and progress of the disease can be predicted.

捏诊:检查者以左手或右手,在患者一定的部位上按捏。

Pinching: The examiner pinches certain positions of the patient with his or her left or right hand.

在按捏时,如发现组织发硬、有抵抗或疼痛等异常变化时,表示有疾病的存在。

During pinching, any abnormal change such as hardening, resisting or aching shows that there is a disease.

(二) 梅花针特定刺激部位全身各部区分布示意图

(Ⅱ) Distribution Diagram of Specially Stimulating Parts of Body for Plum-Blossom Needle

特定刺激部位,是梅花针治病的一个特色。

The specially stimulating part is one of the features of plum-blossom needle therapy.

其刺激部位,是以中医经络学说中十二经所分布的区域为依据。

The stimulating parts are based on the distribution areas of 12 meridians in the TCM theory of meridians and collaterals.

《中国针灸学》提出人体各部分区分为头部、颈部、项部、躯干及四肢穴位的分部法,于梅花针特定刺激部位的划分颇为适用。

The *Chinese Acupuncture and Moxibustion* says that the human body is divided into acupoints of the head, neck, napex, trunk and limbs. This is very suitable to divide the specific stimulating parts of plum-blossom needle.

由于梅花针刺激的范围较广,每一个刺激部位都涉及几条经络之循行部位,包括了许多穴位。

The stimulation scope of plum-blossom needle is wide, and each stimulating part is involved with several meridians and collaterals and many acupoints.

人体各部区之划分(图 1-2、图 1-3),头部位于身体之最上部,分为头盖和颜面部。

The division of human body is shown in Figs. 1-2 and 1-3, and the head on the uppermost part of the body is subdivided into the parts of skull and face.

颈部和项部,为头颅与躯干连接之圆柱状部分,通常分为前颈部、后颈部、左右侧颈部三部分。

The neck and napex, a cylinder-shaped part between the head and trunk, is generally subdivided into parts of anterior neck, posterior neck and lateral neck.

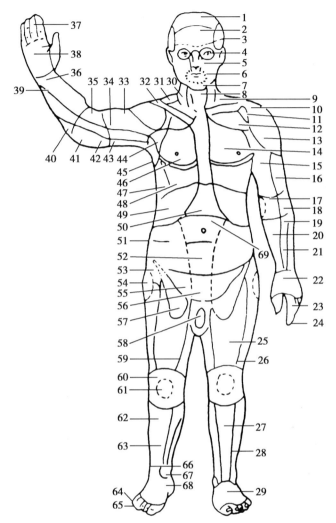

1. 颅顶部；2. 前头部；3. 颞颥部；4. 眶部；5. 鼻部；6. 口部；7. 颐(颌)部；8. 前颈部；9. 颈侧部；
10. 肩胛部；11. 三角胸部；12. 锁骨下部；13. 三角肌部；14. 胸骨部；15. 肱前部；16. 肱外侧
部；17. 肘前部；18. 肘外侧部；19. 桡骨侧臂前部；20. 前臂指掌侧部；21. 前臂背侧部；22. 手
背部；23. 指背部；24. 指部；25. 大腿前部；26. 大腿外侧部；27. 小腿前部；28. 小腿外侧部；
29. 足背部；30. 胸锁乳突肌部；31. 后颈部；32. 锁骨部；33. 肱前部；34. 肱内侧部；35. 肘前
部；36. 前臂掌侧部；37. 指掌侧部；38. 掌侧；39. 前臂尺骨侧部；40. 后肘部；41. 鹰嘴部；
42. 肘内侧部；43. 肱内侧部；44. 腋部；45. 腋窝；46. 乳部；47. 胸侧部；48. 乳下部；49. 季肋
部；50. 上腹部；51. 侧腹部；52. 下腹部；53. 腹股沟部；54. 髋骨部；55. 耻骨部；56. 腹股沟下
部；57. 转子部；58. 外阴部；59. 大腿内侧部；60. 膝前部；61. 膝盖部；62. 小腿前部；63. 小腿
内侧部；64. 趾背部；65. 趾部；66. 内踝后部；67. 内踝部；68. 跟骨部；69. 脐部。

1. Vertex part；2. fore head part；3. temple part；4. orbital part；5. nasal part；6. oral part；
7. zygomatic part；8. anterior neck part；9. lateral neck part；10. scapular part；11. trigonum

pectoralis part; 12. infraclavicular part; 13. deltoid part; 14. sternal part; 15. anterior humeral part; 16. lateral humeral part; 17. anterior elbow part; 18. lateral part of elbow; 19. anterior part of lateral arm of radius; 20. palmar side part of forearm; 21. dorsal side part of forearm; 22. dorsal side part of hand; 23. dorsal part of fingers; 24. digital part of hand; 25. anterior part of thigh; 26. lateral part of thigh; 27. anterior part of lower leg; 28. lateral part of lower leg; 29. dorsal part of foot; 30. sternocleidomastoid part; 31. nape part; 32. clavicular part; 33. anterior part of humerus; 34. medial part of humerus; 35. anterior part of elbow; 36. palmar part of forearm; 37. palmar part of fingers; 38. palm side; 39. lateral part of ulna of forearm; 40. posterior part of elbow; 41. olecranal part; 42. medial part of elbow; 43. medial part of humerus; 44. axillary part; 45. axillary fossa part; 46. mammary part; 47. lateral part of chest; 48. lower part of breast; 49. hypochondriac part; 50. epigastrium; 51. lateral abdomenal part; 52. hypogastrium; 53. inguinal part; 54. hip bone part; 55. pubis part; 56. inferior part of inguen; 57. trochanteric part; 58. vulval part; 59. medial part of thigh; 60. anterior part of knee; 61. knee part; 62. anterior part of lower leg; 63. interior part of lower leg; 64. dorsal part of toe; 65. digital part of foot; 66. posterior part of medial malleolus; 67. medial malleolus part; 68. calcaneal part; 69. umbilical part.

图 1-2　人体前面各部区分布

Fig. 1-2　Distribution of parts in frontal body

躯干分为胸部、腹部和背部。

The trunk is subdivided into parts of chest, abdomen and back.

四肢分上肢部（肱、前臂、手）和下肢部（大腿、小腿、足）。

Limbs are subdivided into parts of upper limbs (upper arms, forearms and hands) and lower limbs (thighs, shanks and feet).

二、梅花针操作技术

Ⅱ. Operation Technique of Plum-Blossom Needle

（一）练针

(I) Training for Needling

为了增强手腕的弹力和力度,术者应掌握正确的叩打手法,这是决定治疗效果的重要环节。

To enhance the flexibility and strength of wrist, the operator should master correct tapping technique, which is an important step to determine the treatment effects.

对不同的疾病和不同的叩打部位,必须采用轻重不同的刺激量。

Stimulation of different qualities must be applied to different diseases or different positions.

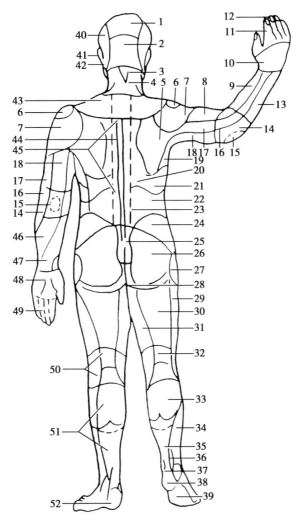

1. 颅顶部；2. 后头部；3. 项窝；4. 项部；5. 肩胛部；6. 肩峰部；7. 三角肌部；8. 肱前部；9. 前臂桡骨侧部；10. 手背部；11. 指背部；12. 指部；13. 前臂背侧部；14. 后肘部；15. 鹰嘴部；16. 肘外（侧）部；17. 肱外侧部；18. 肱后部；19. 胸（外）侧部；20. 肩胛下部；21. 季肋部；22. 腹（外）侧部；23. 腰部；24. 髋骨部；25. 骶骨部；26. 臀部；27. 转子部；28. 会阴部；29. 大腿外（侧）部；30. 大腿后（侧）部；31. 大腿内（侧）部；32. 腘窝；33. 腓肠部；34. 小腿外侧部；35. 小腿后部；36. 外踝后部；37. 外踝部；38. 跟（骨）部；39. 足跖部；40. 颞颥部；41. 耳壳部；42. 乳突部；43. 肩胛上部；44. 肩胛间部；45. 背正中部；46. 前臂尺骨侧部；47. 前臂掌侧部；48. 掌部；49. 指掌侧部；50. 膝后部；51. 小腿后部；52. 跟（骨）部。

1. Epicranial part；2. posterior head；3. nuchal fossa part；4. nuchal part；5. scapular part；6. cromial part；7. deltoid part；8. anterior part of humerus；9. lateral radial part of forearm；10. dorsal part of hand；11. dorsal part of fingers；12. digital part of hand；13. dorsal part of forearm；14. posterior part of elbow；15. olecranal part；16. lateral part of elbow；17. lateral

part of humerus;18. posterior part of humerus;19. lateral part of chest;20. infrascapular part;21. hypochondriac region;22. lateral abdominal part;23. waist part;24. hip bone part; 25. sacral part;26. gluteal part;27. trochanteric part;28. perineal part;29. lateral part of thigh; 30. posterior part of thigh;31. interior part of thigh;32. popliteal fossa part;33. sural part; 34. lateral crus;35. posterior part of lower leg;36. posterior part of lateral malleolus;37. lateral malleolus part;38. calcaneal part;39. metatarsal part;40. temple part;41. tragal part;42. papilla part;43. supscapular part;44. interscapular part;45. middle part of back;46. ulnar part of forearm;47. palmar part of forearm;48. palmar part;49. palmar part of finger;50. posterior part of knee;51. posterior part of lower leg;52. calcaneal part.

图 1-3　人体后面各部区分布

Fig. 1-3　Distribution of parts in posterior body

刺激过重,必将增加患者的痛苦。

Excessive stimulation will increase the patient's pain.

刺激太轻,又不能达到治疗的目的,影响治疗的效果。

Too light stimulation cannot achieve the therapeutic purpose and affect therapeutic effects.

叩打时必须叩平、叩准、叩稳,力度与速度适宜,因此术者必须事前练好手法。

When knocking,the operator must tap flatly,exactly,and steady,and the intensity must match with the speed,so the operator must practice his or her technique in advance.

练针必须做到下列各点:

During training for needling,the following requirements must be followed:

1. 术者用左手握住右手腕,左手再用适当的力量使右手腕关节上下摆动,练习手腕的弹力,或者用右手腕上下弹动,如同西医叩诊一样。

1. The operator should hold right wrist with left hand and make right wrist joints swing up and down with appropriate force to practice the flexibility of wrist or catapult right wrist up and down,just like percussion in Western medicine.

2. 右手持针,可先在枕头等软物上进行叩刺。

2. Hold the needle with the right hand to perform needle tapping on pillows and other soft objects.

其目的一是练习手腕弹力,二是练习叩准、叩稳,以便以后在人体上叩刺。

One of the aims is practicing flexibility of wrist, and the other is tapping exactly and steady, so as to perform needle tapping on human body.

3. 在练习一定的时间后,可在自己手臂或大腿上叩刺,纠正缺点和不正确的手法,以便在患者身上进行治疗。

3. After practicing for some time, the operator can practice needle tapping on his/her own arm or thigh to correct shortcomings and incorrect techniques, so as to provide treatment for patients.

（二）操作前准备

（Ⅱ）Preparation Before Operation

1. 持针 术者用右手握住针柄的尾端,以环指和小指将针柄的尾端固定于手掌小鱼际处,针柄尾端露出手掌 1~1.5cm,再以中指和拇指扶持针柄,示指固定在针柄的前端（中段）,使针不能向四周摆动（图 1-4）。

1. Needle Holding The operator holds the tail end of the needle handle with the right hand, fastens the tail end to hypothenar position in the palm with the ring finger and little finger with the tail end 1-1.5cm above the palm, supports the needle handle with the middle finger and thumb, and put the forefinger on the front end (central section) of the needle handle so as to make the needle unable to swing around (Fig.1-4).

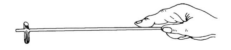

图 1-4 梅花针持针手法

Fig. 1-4 Needle holding skills for Plum-Blossom Needle

将针固定好后,再灵活、适当地运用手腕的弹力和冲力进行叩刺。

After the needle is fixed, the operator performs needle tapping flexibly and properly by using the flexibility and momentum of the wrist.

叩刺时,落针要准、要稳,针尖与皮肤呈垂直接触,提针要快,拔出要有短促清脆的"哒哒"声。

When tapping, the operator should put the needles down exactly and steadily, with the needle points going into the patient's skin vertically, and lift the needles very quickly, and a short and clear sound of "Da, Da..." can be heard.

就这样将针反复提落,连续不断地、有节奏地进行叩刺。

In such a way, needle tapping is performed continuously and rhythmically by repeatedly lifting and lowering the needles.

以上就是弹刺手法的要领,一般每分钟叩打 70~90 次。

The above are main points of technique in needle tapping, and generally 70-90 times of tapping per minute may be done.

2. **解释** 为了取得患者的积极配合,在治疗前应向患者进行必要的解释,包括刺激的疼痛程度、疗程、疾病的预后等,尤其对初诊患者,更加必要,以免患者产生恐惧心理,从而不愿意接受本疗法的治疗,或因不能连续治疗而影响疗效。

2. Explanation To achieve the cooperation of patients, the operator should give necessary explanation to the patients before treatment, including the degree of aching caused by acupuncture, course of treatment and progress of disease. This is more necessary for patients receiving the treatment for the first time, so as to avoid their fear and unwillingness to receive the treatment, or failure to keep a successive course of treatment. As a result, the effect will be influenced.

3. **消毒** 在术前,除对针具消毒外,对针刺部位也应严格地消毒,以免造成感染。

3. Sterilization Before operation, apart from the needles, the acupuncture positions must be strictly sterilized to prevent infection.

由于本疗法刺激的部位较广,刺激较浅,故只需要 75% 的乙醇消毒即可。

Because this therapy has wide range of positions suitable for needle tapping, and the depth of puncture is very shallow, only 75% alcohol is needed for sterilization.

4. **检查针具** 治疗前必须仔细检查针具,如针尖是否整齐,有否弯曲或带钩,合格后方可使用。

4. Needle Examination Before treatment, the operator must examine whether tips of needles are sharp, smooth, bent or free from any hooks, and only the qualified plum-blossom needle can be used.

5. **体位** 指导患者选取适当的体位,以便于治疗。

5. Position   The operator guides the patient to select an adequate position so it is convenient for treatment.

术者自己也要选择适当的操作位置,否则将会影响治疗效果。

Certainly, the operator himself or herself must select an adequate operation position, otherwise it may influence the treatment.

6. **术者的态度**   在治疗过程中,除了仔细询问病史、详细检查及耐心治疗外,术者的态度也起很重要的作用。

6. Operator's Attitude   During the treatment, the operator's attitude plays an important role, in addition to careful inquiry of case history, detailed inspection and patient treatment.

如果施术者态度不严肃,精神不集中,会影响患者情绪,甚至导致治疗中断而影响疗效。

If the operator is unserious and distracted, the patient would be affected and thus might discontinue the treatment.

(三) 施术方法
(Ⅲ) Operation Methods
1. **循经叩刺法**   循经叩刺是沿着经络路线进行叩刺的一种方法。
1. Needle Tapping along Course of Meridians   It is a method that needle tapping is conducted along the course of the meridians and collaterals.

最常用的是任脉、督脉和膀胱经。

The most frequently used are Ren meridian, Du meridian, and Bladder meridian.

任脉循行于身体之前,对全身阴经脉气有总摄、总任的作用,故有“总任诸阴”和“阴脉之海”的说法。

Ren meridian running in the front of the body can govern the qi of all Yin meridians of the body, so it is also called "general control of all Yin meridians" and "the sea of Yin meridians".

又因督脉能调节一身之阳气,五脏六腑的背俞穴皆分布在背腰部的膀胱经,所以其治疗范围颇广。

In addition, Du meridian can adjust the whole body's yang qi, and all back-shu points of the internal organs are distributed over the Bladder meridian of back and waist, so the treatment scope is very wide.

其次，四肢肘膝关节以下的经络，因原穴、络穴、五输穴等特定穴多分布在肘膝关节以下，故可治疗各相应脏腑经络的疾病。

Second, for meridians and collaterals below the elbow and knee joints of arms and legs, such special acupoints as yuan-primary points, luo-connecting points, five-shu points are mostly distributed there, so the diseases of corresponding zang-fu organs and their meridians and collaterals can be treated.

2. 局部叩刺法　即在病变局部叩刺，或在病变局部由外围向中心围刺或散刺。

2. Local Needle Tapping　Needle tapping on the local part of lesion, or surrounded needling or scattered needling from periphery part to center on local part of lesion.

在脊柱两侧及体表其他部位检查，发现阳性物（条索状物、结节状物、海绵状物）及阳性反应区（酸、痛、麻、木）时，治疗中需重点叩打。

Examination is carried out in both sides of spinal column and other positions of body surface. Any positive indicators (strip-like, node-like or sponge-like indicators) and positive reaction area (ache, pain or numbness) detected should be taken as the key parts for needle tapping.

对疼痛或酸痛区的叩打：在此区叩打，必须细心找到最痛的反应点，在痛点皮区做重点叩打，并加用辅助手法，即以左手示指、拇指指尖不时揉按痛点，并向四周疏散揉按。

Needle tapping on aching or paining area: First the most painful reactive points must be found carefully and then on the skin area of the reactive points the major tapping are performed with an auxiliary manipulation, that is the doctor rubs and presses the painful points with his/her tips of forefinger and thumb of left hand, and further rubs and presses the surrounding area.

对麻木皮区的叩打：麻木区的叩打，除对皮肤感觉迟钝或消失的阳性区进行密集叩刺外，还要在麻木区的周围健康皮肤处做疏通性叩打。

Needle tapping on skin area: Intensively, tapping should be performed on the positive areas with insensitivity or numbness. In addition, dredging tapping should be done on the healthy skin surrounding the numb area.

即用梅花针先叩打正常皮肤区,然后逐渐向麻木阳性反应区呈向心性叩打。

That is,tap the normal skin area with the plum-blossom needle first,and then onto the positive reaction area of numbness gradually in a centripetal way.

3. 穴位叩刺法　即在选择好的穴位表面区进行叩刺。

3. Needle Tapping at Acupoints　Needle tapping is performed at selected acupoint in surface area.

临床较常用的有各种特定穴、夹脊穴、阿是穴等。

It is commonly used in all kinds of special acupoints,Jiaji points,Ashi points,etc.

一般以穴位表面 0.5~2cm 为直径做圆形均匀叩刺,每个穴位开始 20 次左右,随后可增至 40~50 次。

Generally speaking,circular and uniformed close tapping is performed on acupoint surface with a diameter of 0.5-2cm,20 times or so for each acupoint firstly and then it may be increased to 40-50 times.

临床治疗方案的确定通常遵循以下三原则:①常规部位、重点部位与局部病变部位相结合的原则;②循经取穴与局部取穴相结合的原则;③经验取穴与常规取穴相结合的原则。

In determination of clinical treatment plan,usually the following three principles should be adhered to:① combining conventional positions,major positions and local lesion positions;② combining acupoint selection based on meridian course with local acupoint selection;③ combining acupoint selection according to experience with acupoint selection based on normal practice.

(四) 施术手法

(Ⅳ) Operation Skills

1. 正刺法　临床最常用。

1. Moderate Tapping　It is the most commonly used in clinic.

就是在叩打时,用力介于轻、重刺法之间,采用既不轻也不重的叩打手法。

The force exerted in the moderate tapping is between that of the light and heavy tapping.

这种手法一般用于常规治疗以及四肢部位。

This kind of tapping is usually applied to normal treatment and four limbs.

2. 轻刺法　为临床常用。

2. Light Tapping　It is commonly used in clinic.

用梅花针在特定的皮肤部位进行轻微叩打,使患者感到微痛。

Light tapping is conducted by exerting a slight force on specific sites of the skin with plum-blossom needle until the patient feels mild pain.

这种手法适用于口、眼、鼻区,头面部,颈部,小儿疾病及久病体弱的患者。

This kind of tapping is suitable for the patients with diseases in mouth, eyes, nose, head, face, neck and pediatric patients, as well as infirm patients with chronic diseases.

3. 重刺法　为临床常用。

3. Heavy Tapping　It is commonly used in clinic.

叩打时用力较"轻刺法"稍重,刺激时有较明显的疼痛,有时也可见肌肉收缩,患者偶尔有躲闪,面部表情有时有变化或有出汗等现象,但要以患者能忍受为度。

Heavy tapping is usually conducted by exerting a little stronger force than "light tapping". Upon operation, the patient may have evident pain, or sometimes have muscle contraction; the patient may occasionally dodge, or have abnormal facial expression, or sweat. However, the operation should be limited to the point of the patient's tolerance.

这种手法多用于胸背部及四肢等部位,一般适用于失去知觉(麻痹)的局部、病体的酸胀部及腰酸背痛、新病体强的患者。

This kind of tapping is usually used on the chest, back and limbs, and generally suitable for a local region with numbness(torpidity), or region with sore or swelling sensation, or with sore waist or backache, or for a strong patient newly suffering from a disease.

4. 平刺法(又名划刺法)　这种手法不用叩打,而是用针尖轻轻地在皮肤上反复滑行刺激,虽然没有疼痛感觉,但是也能起到调整作用。

4. Horizontal Tapping（Also Called Scratching）　It is to make needle tips to repeatedly slide on the skin with gentle force. Actually, it is not a kind of tapping and generally does not induce pain, but it can play a role of regulation.

这种手法适于对针刺很敏感的患者,也可作为重刺激后的配合使用。

This technique is suitable for patients who are sensitive to tapping, and can also for patients who have received heavy tapping.

但划刺的时间应稍长一些。

The time of scratching should generally be a little longer.

5. 放血刺法　对某些特殊的疾病,如高血压等,可用放血刺法。

5. Bleeding Tapping　It can be used for some special diseases, such as hypertension.

在叩打时,术者可用左手捏住刺激的部位,右手持针,用适当的力量叩打,然后用左手在刺激的局部挤压,挤出少量的血液,再用消毒的干棉球擦干局部即可。

The operator can pinch the part to be stimulated with left hand and hold a needle with right hand to do tapping with appropriate force, then squeeze the local stimulated site with left hand to get a little blood out, wipe the local part with sterilized dry cotton ball.

放血的部位,可在颈后区、手指、足趾、鼻尖、下腹部及乳房等处。

The bleeding site can be located at posterior neck, finger, toe, nasal tip, hypogastrium, breast, etc.

6. 强刺法　临床偶尔使用或少用。

6. Strong Tapping　It is occasionally used in clinic.

刺激时疼痛比较明显,患者几乎不能忍受,多数患者有出汗现象。

There comes apparent pain at stimulation, the patients can hardly bear it, and most patients sweat.

多用于感觉迟钝或麻痹的患者。

It is usually suitable for patients with insensitivity and numbness.

7. **超强刺法** 紧急时用。

7. **Ultra-strong Tapping** It is used in emergent situations.

刺激时非常疼痛,患者不能忍受,易晕针。

Serious pain appears at stimulation,the patients cannot bear it and is easy to faint during acupuncture.

多用于急救,如休克、昏迷、癔症或癫痫发作等。

It is usually used in emergency treatment,such as shock,coma,hysteria or epilepsy.

三、临床应用

Ⅲ. Clinical Application

(一) 适应范围

(Ⅰ) Application Range

1. **内科** 头痛、偏头痛、腹痛、胃脘痛、神经麻痹、痉挛、胃及十二指肠溃疡、高血压、冠心病、眩晕、风湿性关节炎、类风湿关节炎、神经衰弱、咳嗽、支气管哮喘、阳痿、早泄等。

1. **In Internal Medicine** Headache,migraine,abdominal pain,epigastric pain,neural paralysis,spasm,gastroduodenal ulcer,hypertension,coronary artery heart disease,vertigo,rheumatic arthritis,rheumatoid arthritis,neurasthenia,cough,bronchial asthma,impotence and premature ejaculation,etc.

2. **骨伤科** 落枕、肌肉扭伤、骨折延期愈合等。

2. **In Osteology and Traumatology** Stiff neck,muscle sprain,delayed union of fracture,etc.

3. **妇科** 月经病、功能失调性子宫出血等。

3. **In Gynecology** Menopathy,dysfunctional uterine bleeding,etc.

4. **儿科** 小儿麻痹后遗症、消化不良、遗尿等。

4. **In Pediatric** Sequelae of polio,dyspepsia,enuresis,etc.

5. **皮肤科** 脱发、神经性皮炎、丹毒、多汗症、皮肤瘙痒症、斑秃等。

5. **In Dermatology** Alopecia,neurodermatitis,erysipelas,hyperhidrosis,

cutaneous pruritus,alopecia areata,etc.

6. **外科**　淋巴结炎、淋巴结核、腱鞘炎、某些手术后遗症、尿潴留等。

6. **In Surgery**　Lymphadenitis,lymphadenoid tuberculosis,tenosynovitis,surgical sequelae,urinary retention,etc.

7. **耳鼻喉科**　鼻炎、感觉神经性耳聋、牙痛、屈光不正、睑腺炎、视神经萎缩等。

7. **In Otorhinolaryngology**　Rhinitis,sensorineural deafness,toothache,ametropia,hordeolum,optic atrophy,etc.

(二) 处方示例

(Ⅱ) Prescription Examples

1. 高血压

1. Hypertension

（1）配方一:重点刺激第 1~5 胸椎及其两侧与检查发现的异常部位。

（1）Prescription 1:The 1st-5th thoracic vertebrae and the two sides of them as well as abnormal sites detected by examination are mainly stimulated.

采用轻刺法和正刺法。

Light tapping and moderate tapping are adopted.

先叩刺脊柱两侧 3 行 2 遍,再重点刺激第 1~5 胸椎及其两侧与检查发现的异常部位 5 行 5 遍,然后对上腹部、前后肋间区和病变部位做局部刺激。

Both sides of the spine are firstly tapped by three rows for two times,1st-5th thoracic vertebrae and their sides are tapped by five rows for five times,then abnormal sites are tapped,finally,the upper abdomen and anterior and posterior intercostal regions are locally tapped.

每日叩打 1 次,10 次为 1 个疗程。

Tapping is conducted once every day,10 times for one course.

（2）配方二:血压在 200~220/120~130mmHg 者,取颈部前后、骶部、耳甲、外耳道及耳后之乳突部、头顶部。

（2）Prescription 2:For the patients with blood pressure of 200-220/120-130 mmHg,the anterior and posterior neck,sacral part,auricular concha,external auditory meatus, mastoid process at posterior ear and vertical part are tapped.

采用轻刺法、正刺法或重刺法。

Light tapping, moderate tapping or heavy tapping is adopted.

先轻刺骶部,休息数分钟后,再中度(正刺)刺激颈后部,休息一下,重刺颈前部、中刺耳甲、耳后之乳突部,再轻刺头顶部。

Light tapping is firstly conducted on the sacral part, several minutes later, moderate tapping is conducted on the posterior neck. After a rest, heavy tapping is conducted on the anterior neck, and moderate tapping is applied on the auricular concha and mastoid process at posterior ear. Finally, light tapping is applied on vertical part.

每日叩打 1 次。

Tapping is conducted once every day.

2. 便秘

2. Constipation

(1) 配方一:取脊柱两侧、下腹部、脐周围区、腰骶部及其两侧。

(1) Prescription 1:Both sides of the spine, the hypogastrium, the part surrounding the umbilicus, the lumbosacral parts and their sides.

采用轻刺法或正刺法。

Light tapping or moderate tapping is adopted.

先叩刺脊柱两侧3行1或2遍,再重点刺激腰骶部及其两侧5行各4~5遍,然后对下腹部、脐周围区做局部刺激。

Both sides of the spine are tapped by 3 rows for 1 or 2 times, lumbosacral parts and their sides are tapped by 5 rows for 4-5 times, and then hypogastrium and part surrounding the umbilicus are locally tapped.

每日叩打 1 次,至大便正常为度。

Tapping is conducted once every day until stool can be discharged normally.

(2) 配方二:顽固性便秘(肠狭窄)取脊柱两侧、下腹部(脐眼直下之中线和双侧天枢直下之侧线)、下肢外侧区、腰骶部及其两侧。

(2) Prescription 2:For obstipation(intestinal stenosis), the both sides of

spine, the hypogastrium (the midline downright from the umbilicus and lateral line downright from Tianshu of both sides), the lateral regions of lower limbs, the lumbosacral parts and their sides should be operated.

采用轻刺法或正刺法。

Light tapping or moderate tapping is adopted.

先叩刺脊柱两侧3行各3遍，再重点刺激腰骶部及其两侧5行各往返3次，后对下腹部、下肢外侧区做局部刺激往返3次。

Both sides of spine are tapped by 3 rows for 3 times, the lumbosacral parts and their sides are tapped by 5 rows for 3 times, and then the hypogastrium and lateral regions of lower limbs are locally tapped for 3 times.

每日叩打1次，持续1个月。

Tapping is conducted once every day, for a successive month.

3. 癃闭
3. Retention of Urine

取脊柱两侧，并重点叩刺第1~3胸椎或第11~12胸椎，或腰骶椎及其两侧，下腹部正中线（任脉）、腘窝处、肺俞、脾俞、肾俞、三焦俞、膀胱俞、中极。

Both sides of the spine, particularly 1st-3th thoracic vertebrae or 11th-12th thoracic vertebrae, or lumbosacral vertebrae and their sides, median line of hypogastrium (Ren meridian), popliteal fossa, Feishu, Pishu, Shenshu, Sanjiaoshu, Pangguangshu, Zhongji are tapped.

采用正刺法。

Moderate tapping is adopted.

对所选部位和穴位施以中度手法叩刺3~5行（重点区为5行），每穴20~30下，至皮肤出现潮红，微见出血为度。

Moderate tapping is conducted on selected sites and acupoints by 3-5 rows (5 rows in major areas), 20-30 times for each acupoint, till skin is flushed with slight bleeding.

叩刺后指压"利尿穴"（神阙至曲骨连线的中点即是），并逐渐加大力度，压到一定程度即可排尿，继续按压至尿完全排出为止。

After tapping，"Diuretic acupoint"（the midpoint of Shenque to Qugu line）is pressed with finger, and as force is gradually increased, urine can be discharged. Do not stop pressing till urine is fully discharged.

每日叩打 1 次，中病即止。

Tapping is performed once per day and discontinued as soon as it gets effect.

（三）禁忌证

（Ⅲ）Contraindications

1. 凡是外伤、难产、急腹症、急性出血、诊断未明确的高热和急性传染病、严重器质性疾病、重度贫血、严重心脏病、癌症晚期及叩刺后容易引起出血的疾病，应列为禁忌证。

1. Contraindications include trauma, dystocia, acute abdomen disease, acute bleeding, high fever with no clear diagnosis and acute infectious disease, severe organic disease, severe anemia, serious heart disease, terminal cancer and other diseases which can result in bleeding after tapping.

2. 下列情况也应慎用，如咯血、呕血、尿血、便血和外伤性大出血疾病，应避免叩刺出血部位，以防叩刺后加重出血。

2. For hemoptysis, hematemesis, hematuria, hematochezia and traumatic hemorrhage diseases, tapping should be cautiously used. Tapping cannot be applied on bleeding sites to prevent worsening bleeding.

3. 各种骨折，忌在患部叩刺，可在患部附近用轻手法叩刺。

3. Tapping on fractured sites should be avoided, while light tapping can be conducted near fractured sites.

4. 妇女怀孕期间应慎用。

4. For women who are in pregnancy, tapping should be cautiously used.

5. 各种皮肤病、疖肿、皮肤感染，不宜在患部叩刺。

5. For dermatosis, furuncles and skin infection, tapping on affected sites should be avoided.

（四）注意事项

（Ⅳ）Precautions

1. 治疗前应详细询问病史，仔细检查，必要时应配合理化检查，求得较明确的诊断,这既有利于治疗,又便于今后总结及避免医疗事故的发生。

1. Before treatment, medical history should be carefully inquired about and examinations should be carefully conducted, and physicochemical examination can be taken to get clearer diagnosis, which is beneficial to treatment, and can facilitate future summary and avoid occurrence of medical accidents.

2. 术前需要患者稍微休息,一般休息 10 分钟即可,消除紧张情绪,使全身肌肉放松,方可施治。

2. Before treatment, patients should have a rest, generally for 10 minutes, to remove their nervousness and make the whole-body muscle relaxed, and then treatment can be conducted.

否则可能会因情绪紧张、肌肉不放松而影响治疗效果,疲劳过度的患者也不要立即施治,要先休息,恢复常态后再予施治。

Otherwise treatment effects will be affected due to emotional tension and unrelaxed muscle. The overtired patients should have a rest first, and then receive treatment.

3. 要根据患者体质、性别、年龄和神经型与非神经型及疾病的病情不同等情况来选择最佳的叩刺手法。

3. The tapping techniques should be appropriately selected according to the patients' constitution, gender, age, pathological state and different conditions of disease.

4. 根据治疗方案确定刺激部位。

4. The stimulating parts should be determined based on the treatment plan.

施治时,刺激部位和面积不宜过多过大,对于过多的刺激部位、过大的刺激面积可适当配合,轮换使用,不必一次全用。

During treatment, the stimulating parts should not be too many and the areas should not be too large. All stimulating parts or areas where the operation should be applied can be conducted coordinately and alternately, but not necessarily selected in one time.

5. 术时要注意室内环境和气温,避开风口,以免因受凉而加重病情,影响治疗。

5. During operation, indoor environment and temperature should be noted. Operation should not be conducted at windy places to avoid catching cold to worsen the condition and affect the effect.

有些疾病如高血压,应在安静的室内进行治疗,以免影响患者的情绪,而影响治疗效果。

For some diseases like hypertension, the patients should be treated in a quiet room so as not to affect the patient's emotions and treatment efficacy.

6. 根据病情的轻重缓急,注意在治疗过程中的间隔及疗程,注意观察有效的刺激部位,同时在病历和病情记录上应尽量详细记录。

6. According to the disease severity and emergency degree, interval and treatment course should be noted during the treatment, and effective stimulating parts should be observed. Meanwhile, relevant information should be recorded in medical cases and disease progress.

7. 叩刺部位的皮肤和针具,术前要进行常规消毒,以防感染。

7. The skin to be tapped and the needles to be used should be sterilized before treatment to prevent infection.

同时术前要检查针具,针尖必须平齐、无弯钩、无锈蚀。

The operator must examine whether tips of needles are sharp, smooth, and free from any hooks and rustiness.

8. 初次接受治疗的患者和小儿,宜用轻刺法,以后再根据病情逐渐加重。

8. For patients and children receiving treatment for the first time, light tapping should be applied, and then other tapping techniques can be adopted according to the condition of disease.

9. 在施治时,要关心患者,要严肃认真地小心操作,切忌麻痹大意,并随时询问患者的感觉,如发现异常情况,应及时变换叩刺手法或中止治疗进行观察,并加以必要的处理。

9. During treatment, the operator should care for patients and implement treatment strictly and carefully, carelessness should be avoided, and patient's feeling should be inquired about at any time. In case of any abnormal situation, tapping technique should be changed in time or treatment should be stopped for

observation, and necessary treatment should be implemented.

10. 叩刺时,要注意按叩刺方向和顺序进行,以免倒置或疏密不均。

10. Tapping should be conducted in a given direction and sequence so as to avoid inversion or uneven density.

叩刺后,应嘱患者休息数分钟后再走,以免在返家途中发生意外。

After tapping, the patient should first have a rest for several minutes to prevent occurrence of accidents when returning home.

11. 手法快慢、刺激强度要根据病情、体质和叩刺部位而决定。

11. Tapping speed and intensity should be determined according to the patients' disease conditions, constitution and tapping sites.

一般用轻刺法或正刺法,以皮肤没有红晕或以不出血为宜。

Generally speaking, light tapping or moderate tapping should be adopted, and cause no skin blushing or bleeding.

用重刺法时,应以轻微出血为度。

Heavy tapping should be conducted until slight bleeding occurs.

对于体质虚弱、贫血及有心脏病的患者,操作手法要快些、轻些。

For patients with weak constitution, anemia and heart diseases, tapping should be quickly and slightly conducted.

初诊时叩刺面积不应太大,以后逐渐增加面积。

Tapping area for the first time should not be too large, and then it can be gradually increased.

12. 对久治不愈的患者,应研究刺激的部位、强度、间隔时间等情况是否恰当,必要时可配合其他疗法或会诊,制定新的治疗方案,以免延误患者的治疗。

12. For patients without obvious improvement after the treatment, the doctor should research whether stimulating parts, intensity and intervals are proper, and formulate new treatment plan by combining other therapy or through consultation so as not to delay the treatment.

13. 在治疗时,应注意患者与术者体位的配合,否则将会影响治疗的效果,妨碍叩刺操作的发挥,同时也给患者治疗带来不必要的影响。

13. During the treatment, the postures of the patient and operator should be coordinated, otherwise efficacy may be affected, the tapping cannot be normally conducted, and unnecessary influence will be brought to the patient.

患者体位既要舒适，又要便于操作。

The posture of the patient should be comfortable and facilitate the treatment.

（五）意外的处理方法

（Ⅴ）Treatment for Accidents

1. 晕针的处理　在叩刺过程中，如患者感到头晕、眼花，出冷汗，严重时面色苍白、脉搏微细、手脚发凉，甚至晕倒，考虑晕针发生，应立即停止针刺，让患者平卧休息，并给予温开水或糖水，严重者予以吸氧、补液等急救措施。

1. Treatment of Fainting During Acupuncture　If the patient has symptoms of dizziness, blurred vision, cold sweat, even pale face, weak and thread pulse, cold hands and feet and fall in a faint during tapping, fainting during acupuncture is considered. At this time, acupuncture should be stopped immediately, and let the patient lie in supine position, give him/her warm boiled water or sugar water, and such emergency treatment as oxygen inhalation and fluid infusion should be given to severe patients.

2. 头痛、失眠、食欲减退的处理　经过3~5次的针刺后，患者可能出现头痛、失眠、食欲减退的现象，应向患者做必要的解释，并注意刺激间隔时间不要过短，避免手法过强及刺激部位过多。

2. Treatment of Headache, Insomnia and Anorexia　After tapping for 3-5 times, the patient may possibly have headache, insomnia and anorexia, and the operator should give necessary descriptions to the patient, and tapping intervals should not be too short to avoid strong force and excessive stimulating parts.

3. 过敏反应的处理　经过3~5次的针刺后，可能在刺激局部出现皮肤丘疹、发痒等过敏现象，这对身体并无明显影响。

3. Treatment of Allergy　After tapping for 3-5 times, papulae, itching and other allergies may possibly appear at the locally stimulated skin, which has no apparent influence on the body.

故应向患者做必要解释，或嘱患者休息数日后再行针，过敏反应严重者应停止治疗。

Nevertheless, the doctor should give necessary descriptions to the patient, and ask them to have a rest for several days, then the operation can be done further. The operation should be stopped immediately for patients with severe allergy.

4. 血肿的处理　少量的皮下出血或局部小块青紫,一般不必处理,可自行消退。

4. Treatment of Hematoma　A small amount of subcutaneous hemorrhage or local small pieces of cyanosis are not necessarily to be treated, generally they can disappear automatically.

若局部肿胀疼痛较剧,青紫面积大,可先做冷敷 24~48 小时,再做热敷,以促进局部血肿消散吸收。

For the conditions of local swelling, pain and large cyanosis area, cold compressing can be implemented for 20-48 hours first, and then hot compressing so as to promote local hematoma dissipation and absorption.

参 考 文 献
References

[1] 程爵棠. 梅花针疗法治百病[M].5 版. 北京:人民军医出版社,2015.
[2] 曲晖. 梅花针疗法[M]. 北京:金盾出版社,2013.
[3] 申永寿,黄亮,裴巍. 梅花针治百病[M]. 北京:科学技术文献出版社,2009.

第三节　火　　针
Section 3　Fire Needle

火针疗法是用特制的粗针,用火或电将针尖烧红后迅速刺入穴位内以治疗疾病的方法。

Fire needle therapy is to rapidly insert thick needle whose point turns red after burned with fire or electricity into acupoints to treat diseases.

火针疗法具有针和灸的双重作用,通过火针刺激腧穴,其温热作用能增加人体阳气,调节脏腑功能,使经络通畅,气血通行。

Fire needle therapy has dual functions of needling and moxibustion, which can increase yang qi of human body, regulate functions of zang-fu organs, dredge meridians and collaterals, and smooth circulation of qi and blood by warming function resulting from stimulation by fire needle to acupoint.

此外,火针疗法具有祛寒除湿、散结解毒、祛腐排脓、生肌敛疮、益肾壮阳、温中和胃、升阳举陷、宣肺平喘、消肿止痛、息风定惊等作用。

In addition, fire needle therapy has the functions of dispelling coldness and removing dampness, eliminating stagnation and resolving toxin, removing necrotic tissue and evacuating pus, promoting granulation and wound healing, tonifying the kidney and strengthening the yang, warming the spleen and harmonizing the stomach, elevating to cure prolapse and yang qi, ventilating the lung to relieve dyspnea, reducing swelling and alleviating pain, relieving dizziness and arresting convulsion, etc.

火针针具应具有耐高温、坚硬挺拔的特点。

Needling instruments of fire needle therapy are characteristically high temperature resistant and hard.

火针一般取 26 或 27 号 1.5~2.5 寸不锈钢毫针。

For fire needle therapy, generally No.26 or No.27 and 1.5-2.5 cun stainless steel filiform needle is used.

直径为 0.5mm 的细火针主要用于小儿或体弱者。

Thin fire needle with 0.5mm diameter is mainly used for children or patients with weak condition.

直径为 1.0mm 的火针,适用范围比较广泛,除面部穴位和肌肉较薄的部位外,其他四肢躯干、压痛点和病灶四周均可应用。粗火针直径为 2.0~2.5mm。

The fire needle with 1.0mm diameter has a broad scope of application and can be used in the four limbs and trunk, tenderness point and the position around nidus besides facial acupoints and the body part with less muscle. The thick fire needle generally has a diameter of 2.0-2.5mm.

火针针柄多用竹或骨质包裹,以免烫手。

The handle of fire needle is often covered with bamboo or sclerotin to avoid burning hands.

用于浅刺的,针身比较细短,装在一个木制柄上,便于叩刺,也可在针柄上同时装 3~9 枚钢针,以加强刺激,形状与梅花针相似。

The fire needle used for shallow needling has a thin and short needle body and is mounted on a wooden handle for needle tapping. The needle handle may also be provided with 3-9 steel needles that have the same shape as that of plum-blossom needle to reinforce stimulation.

近年来,针灸学者们根据临床需要研制出了多种类型电火针,如高频感应加热火针、直流电火针等,这些新型电火针由于在携带和操作上都非常方便、简洁,所以被广泛应用于临床。

In recent years, acupuncture scholars have developed multiple types of electrical fire needles according to clinical requirements, such as high frequency induction heating fire needle, DC fire needle, and the like. These new electrical fire needles are widely used in clinic because of simple operation and convenient carrying.

一、火针的选穴原则

Ⅰ. Acupoint Selection Principle of Fire Needle

根据病证不同而辨证选穴。

According to different diseases, select acupoints based on syndrome differentiation.

一般取病变局部穴位或阿是穴,也可邻近取穴、循经取穴,取穴宜少。

Generally, the acupoints on the local part of lesion or Ashi points should be selected, nearby acupoints and acupoints along the meridians may also be selected, and it is appropriate to select a small amount of acupoints.

实证和青壮年患者,取穴可略多。

For the patient with excess syndrome or young adult patients, select a little more acupoints.

火针取穴规律,一般先上后下,先背后腹,先左后右。

Acupoint selection of the fire needle therapy is generally from the top to the bottom, from back to abdomen and from left to right.

在特殊情况下,可以灵活运用。

In a particular case, the selection may be made flexibly.

每次可选 4~6 个穴位,亦可在疗程内拟两组穴交替使用。

Select 4-6 acupoints for each time and alternately use two sets of acupoints in a course of treatment.

(一) 近部取穴
近部取穴是指在病变的局部或临近部位选取腧穴。

(Ⅰ) Nearby Acupoint Selection

This is to select acupoint on the local part of lesion or the position adjacent to the lesion region.

1. **阿是穴**　以痛点为穴位,这类穴位一般都随病而定,没有固定的位置和名称,以局部压痛点来定穴位。

1. **Ashi Points**　Select the pain points as the acupoints. Such acupoints should be determined according to the condition of diseases and have no fixed positions and names. Select the point of local tenderness as acupoint.

2. **病变部位取穴**　病变部位主要指肿块、疮疡、筋瘤、皮损等部位。

2. **Selecting Acupoint in Lesion Region**　The lesion region mainly refers to the location of mass, sore and ulcer, nodular varicosity and skin lesion.

(二) 辨经取穴

(Ⅱ) Acupoint Selection Based on Meridian Differentiation

1. **经脉循行取穴**　紧密结合经脉的循行取穴,体现了"经脉所过、主治所及"的治疗规律。

1. **Acupoint Selection Based on Meridian Course**　Select acupoints entirely in accordance with the running course of the meridians, which reflects the treatment rules of "the parts where the meridians pass should be taken as the major sites of treatment".

2. **标本根结法取穴**　标本根结法取穴是一种特殊的辨经取穴方法,依据标本、根结的理论,选取相关经脉的"根""结"部位。

2. **Acupoint Selection Based on Biao-Ben and Root-Knot**　This is a

special method for acupoint selection based on meridian identification, which selects "root" and "knot" positions of relevant affected meridians according to the theory of Biao (the secondary) -Ben (the primary), and Root-Knot.

3. **辨症取穴** 根据患者最明显的症状或体征,选取相应的穴位,多取不同经脉上的原穴治疗。

3. **Acupoint Selection Based on Symptom Differentiation** Select corresponding acupoints according to the most evident symptom or sign of the patient, generally selecting Yuan (source) acupoint on different meridians for treatment.

4. **辨证取穴** 针对某些全身症状或疾病的病因病机而选取穴位。

4. **Acupoint Selection Based on Syndrome Differentiation** Select acupoints in accordance with the etiology and pathogenesis of certain general symptoms or diseases.

5. **神经节段分布取穴** 相应的内脏和躯体,形成穴位-经络-内脏间的实质联系,故按神经节段分布选取相应穴位,如脊神经的节段性分布。

5. **Acupoint Selection by Nerve Segment Distribution** Corresponding viscera and body form substantial relationship among acupoints, meridians, collaterals and viscera, so select corresponding acupoints according to nerve segment distribution, such as segmental distribution of spinal nerve.

二、火针操作技术

Ⅱ. Operation Techniques of Fire Needle

(一) 操作前准备

(Ⅰ) Preparation Before Operation

1. **选择体位** 根据刺烙点的不同及患者的体质,选择适当的体位。

1. **Selection of Patient's Position** Select appropriate position according to different pricking points and constitution of patients.

常用的有仰卧位、侧卧位、俯卧位、背靠坐位、俯坐位等。

Common positions taken by patients include supine position, lateral position, prone position, sitting position against the backrest, prone sitting position, etc.

一般以便于施术者取穴、操作方便、刺烙点定位后不易偏移和患者舒适的体位为宜,对年老、小儿、体弱者,宜采用卧位或背靠坐位。

The preferable position should be convenient for operator to select acupoints and easy to operate, and again in this position, pricking points cannot easily deviate after they are selected and the patient feels comfortable. It is appropriate for the elderly, children and weak patients to adopt lying position or sitting position against the backrest.

2. 定位　由于火针治疗多进针迅速,故宜事先对选择的穴位或者刺烙点进行定位,并加以标记,以确保针刺的准确性。

2. Locating Position　Because of rapid needling of fire needle treatment, it is appropriate to locate and mark the position of selected acupoint or pricking points in advance, so as to get the accuracy of the acupuncture.

定位采用指甲掐"十"字法,进针点在交叉点,如果刺烙部位为囊肿、脓肿、包块等,可请助手协助固定肿物,以防肿物活动而导致进针点偏移,伤及周围组织。

Locating the position is conducted by pinching the skin with nails to form a "Cross", needling point being the intersection. If pricking position is cyst, abscess, mass and the like, let an assistant fix the lump to prevent it from moving, thereby avoiding deviation of needling point and injuring surrounding tissue.

如果进针点为活动性痛点,则宜请助手协助固定患者体位后再做标记、针刺。

If needling point is an active pain point, it is appropriate to let an assistant mark the point and then to do needing after fixing patient's position.

3. 消毒　定位后,可以用2%~5%碘酒从穴位中心向四周做同心圆消毒,再以75%的酒精棉球同法脱碘。

3. Sterilization　After fixing the position, perform sterilization concentrically from acupoint center to the surrounding area with 2%-5% iodine tincture and then perform deiodination in the same way with 75% alcohol cotton.

若刺烙部位为黏膜或溃疡,则宜用刺激性小的消毒液进行消毒。

If pricking position is mucosa or ulcer, it is appropriate to use bland disinfectant for sterilization.

4. 加热针体　即烧针。

4. Heating Needle Body　Burning the needle.

左手持点燃的酒精灯或95%的酒精棉球于胸前,尽量接近要刺烙的部位,右手拇指、示指、中指微曲夹持针柄,针尖指向进针点,置于灯焰外焰上灼烧,先加热针体,再加热针尖,根据治疗目的的不同可将针烧至白亮、微红、通红3种热度,加热到所需温度后,即可对患处施针。

Hold the ignited alcohol burner or 95% alcohol cotton with the left hand in front of the operator's chest, make them as close as possible to the pricking points, and grip the needle handle with slightly bent thumb, forefinger and middle finger of the right hand to keep the point of a needle pointing to the needling point. Burn the needle with outer flame of the lamp, first heat the needle body and then burn the point of the needle. Burn the needle to three degrees of heat (bright, slight red and very red) according to different therapeutic purposes, and perform acupuncture on the affected part when the needle is heated to required temperature.

(二) 施术方法

(Ⅱ) Operation Methods

火针疗法的手法可以简单概括为:揣、爪、烧、刺、退五个字。

The technique of fire needle therapy can be summarized as five words: Stroking, seizing, burning, piercing and withdrawing.

揣,即是根据病情,沿一定的经络走行进行揣摸,寻找压痛点,"以痛为腧",在揣的过程中要遵循"宁失其穴,勿失其经"的原则。

Stroking, that is, stroke along the running course of certain meridians and collaterals according to patient's condition for seeking tenderness points, "taking the tender point as acupoint", the principle of "one would rather miss the acupoint than miss the meridian" in stroking.

爪,即是以爪甲在所取穴位上按压出痕边,然后用甲紫进行标记。

Seizing, that is, press out a trace on the selected acupoint by fingernail, and mark the trace with gentian violet.

烧,即烧热针,亦即加热针体,使针体达到"通红"的温度。

Burning, that is, heat the needle body, heating it to the degree of "very red".

刺,即将火针迅速准确刺入所标记的腧穴。

Piercing, that is, rapidly pierce the fire needle into the marked acupoint.

退,即拔针,要求必须"速进疾出",因留之过久会致患者痛苦加重。

Withdrawing, that is, withdraw the needle, which requires "quick insertion and withdrawal of the needle", because the patients will feel more painful if the needle retaining time is too long.

操作中,一般所取部位需反复揣按,力求准确,便于火针准确刺入腧穴。

The selected position needs to be stroked and pressed repeatedly to ensure accuracy during operation, so that the fire needle can accurately go into the acupoint.

进针时使针体快速垂直刺入腧穴。

Quickly and vertically insert the needle body into the acupoint when needling.

刺入机体的深度要根据病情轻重、体质与季节不同而定。

The depth of needling depends on patient's condition and constitution as well as season.

出针要疾速,整个针刺过程要做到稳、准、快。

Needle withdrawal should be rapid and the whole operation process should be steady, accurate and rapid.

1. 进针方法

1. Needling Method

（1）点刺法:点刺法是最常用的火针刺法,即将火针烧到所需温度后迅速刺入选定穴位的方法。

（1）Point-pricking: It is the most commonly used fire needle therapy, the method is inserting fire needle quickly into the selected acupoint after the needles are burned to required temperature.

其他火针刺法多以点刺法为基本,只是针刺的深度、密度等有所不同。

All the other methods for fire needle therapy are mainly based on point-pricking, being different only in depth and density of needling.

点刺法多用于缓解疼痛及全身病症。

Point-pricking is mainly used to relieve pain and general symptoms of diseases.

(2) 密刺法：密刺法是用火针密集地刺激病变局部的一种刺法，针刺间隔一般为 1cm 左右，病情重者可相应的密刺。

(2) Dense Needling：It is to compactly stimulate the local part of lesion by using fire needles generally with a spacing about 1 cm. Nevertheless, for a patient with serious condition, a relatively denser needling can be conducted.

针刺深度以针尖透过皮肤病变组织，刚好接触正常组织为宜，故宜根据皮肤厚薄及角质层的硬度来选择针具，皮肤厚硬处宜选用粗火针，反之亦然。

The appropriate depth of needling is that the point of needle just contacts normal tissue after piercing the lesioned tissue of skin. So, needling instrument should be selected according to the thickness of skin and the hardness of cuticle. So the thick fire needle should be used to the thick and hard part of skin, and vice versa.

密刺法可在病变局部蕴积足够的热力，使气血流通，促进组织的再生和修复。

Dense needling can store enough heat in the local part of lesion for promoting a circulation of qi-blood, and regeneration and repair of tissue.

多用于增生性及角化性皮肤病变，如神经性皮炎等。

The therapy is mainly used for treating proliferating and keratinizing skin lesion, such as neurodermatitis.

(3) 围刺法：围刺法是火针围绕病变部位周围进行针刺的方法。

(3) Encircling Needling：This is to insert fire needles around the lesion regions.

一般选用中粗火针，针刺间隔 1~1.5cm 为宜。

The therapy often adopts medium or thick fire needles with a spacing of 1-1.5cm.

对于局部红肿热痛者，可直接用火针刺络放血，此法可改善局部血液循环，可用于臁疮、带状疱疹等。

For the patient with local redness, swelling, hotness and pain, blood-letting by collateral pricking can be conducted directly by fire needles. The therapy can improve local blood circulation and can be used to treat ecthyma, herpes zoster, etc.

（4）散刺法：散刺法是以火针松散地点刺病变部位的针刺方法。

（4）Scattered Needling: This is to insert fire needles in the lesion regions in scattered way.

一般选择细火针，每隔 1.5cm 一针，以浅刺为宜。

The therapy generally adopts thin fire needle with a needling spacing of 1.5cm, and it is advisable to do shallow needling.

此法可以疏通局部气血，具有除痹止痒、解痉止痛的功用，可用于治疗四肢麻木、躯体痛痒、肢体拘挛、疼痛等病症。

The therapy can promote local flow of qi and blood, has the functions of relieving obstruction and relieving itching, relieving spasm and pain. It may be used to treat limbs anesthesia, body pain and itching, limbs contracture and pain, etc.

（5）烙烫法：在施术部位表面轻而缓慢地烙烫，多用平头针，可以治疗色素痣、老年斑、白癜风等疾病，或者赘生物中体积较小者。

（5）Cauterization: This is to lightly and slowly cauterize the surface of operated position with flat-ended needle, which may treat the diseases such as nevus pigmentosus, age pigment and vitiligo or smaller neoplasms.

此法针头与皮肤接触的面积较大，停留时间长，所以患者疼痛尤甚，可以在局部麻醉下进行。

In this therapy, the needle head has a larger area of contact with the skin for a long time, so the patients feel more painful. It can be conducted under local anaesthesia.

（6）割治法：割治法多用粗火针，烧针至所需热度，将火针刺入选定的囊腔低垂部，深度以穿透囊腔为度，出针时摇大针孔，出针后可按压囊腔，务必令囊腔脓液、瘀血、水液等尽出。

（6）Cutting: This is to generally use thick fire needle, burn the needle to the required degree of heat, and insert it into the dropping part of the selected bursal lumen to the extent that the bursal lumen is penetrated. When withdrawing the needle, shake and expand the acupuncture hole, and press the bursal lumen after needle withdrawal to drain pus, stagnated blood, and liquid from the bursal lumen.

如治疗某些皮肤赘生物,常可将灯火放在一旁,用左手持镊子等夹持皮赘等,烧针后,灼烙割切皮赘根部,以切断为度,注意动作不要太快,以免出血,一般一针即好。

For skin neoplasm treatment, put the lights aside and clamp skin tag with tweezers held by the left hand. After burning the needle, cauterize and cut the root of skin tag off. Do not move too fast to avoid bleeding, and one time of operation can affect a cure.

如伤口有渗血,可用平头火针烙熨止血。因割治疗法创伤相对较大,要防止术后感染。

If the wound extravasates, cauterization with flat-ended fire needle is conducted to stop bleeding. The postoperative infection should be prevented because of relatively large wound in this therapy.

如赘生物较多,可分批分次治疗。

If there are more neoplasms, treatment can be performed in batches.

(7) 快针法:进针达合适深度后迅速将针提出,整个过程只有十分之一秒左右。

(7) Quick Needling: This is to rapidly withdraw the needle after appropriate needling depth is reached, and the whole process lasts for one-tenth second or so.

根据进针的深度又可分为深刺速刺、浅点刺等,此法进针出针速度快,往往还未达到形成痛阈的时间,操作已结束,所以疼痛很轻或无疼痛。

The technique can be divided into deep needling and rapid needling and shallow point needling. The speed of insertion and withdrawal of the needle is so quick that operation is completed before reaching the threshold of pain, so the patient feels very little pain or no pain.

操作结束后局部常有灼热感,有时还向远端放射。

After the operation, the patient usually has a burning sensation in local skin, and the sensation sometimes radiates to the far-end.

此法具有温阳散寒、激发经气、行气活血的作用。快针法是火针最常用的方法之一。

The therapy has the functions of warming yang and eliminating cold, exciting meridian qi, activating qi and promoting blood circulation. It is one of the most common method in fire needle therapy.

（8）慢针法：慢针法又称留针刺，是快速将火针刺入一定深度后，逗留一段时间，然后再出针的方法，留针时间多在 1~5 分钟，在留针期间，可行捻转、提插等手法加强针感。

(8) Slow Needling: It is also known as retaining needling, which is to insert the fire needle to a certain depth, make the needle stay at the point for a period of time and withdraw the needle. The needle retaining time is 1-5 minutes, during this period, needling sensation can be strengthened by techniques such as twirling of needle, lifting and thrusting of needle, etc.

此法针感除局部灼热感外，常有酸麻胀感等，具有祛腐化痰、软坚散结的作用。

In addition to local burning sensation, the patient often feels soreness, numbness and distension during acupuncture. The therapy has the functions of removing the necrotic tissue and reducing phlegm, and softening and dissipating hardness.

此法主要用于顽固性疾患、剧痛之疾，如三叉神经痛、顽固的坐骨神经痛、久泻久痢、哮喘频发、神经纤维瘤、风寒久痹、冷痛难愈的肩凝症、慢性盆腔炎、囊肿等疾病。

Slow needling is mainly used to treat intractable diseases and the diseases with severe pain, such as trigeminal neuralgia, intractable sciatica, prolonged diarrhea and dysentery, frequent onset of asthma, neurofibroma, wind-cold-dampness arthralgia, refractory frozen shoulder with crymodynia, chronic pelvic inflammatory disease and cyst, etc.

2. 进针角度　进针的角度为垂直刺入，对赘生物等可采用斜刺法、钩刺法等。

2. Needling Angle　Needling angle is vertical, and oblique needling and hooking needling are applicable for neoplasm.

3. 进针深度　进针的深度视针刺部位、病情性质、患者体质情况及季节气候等多方面因素而定。

3. Needling Depth　The needling depth depends on various factors, such as acupuncture position, nature of patient's condition, patient constitution, season and climate, etc.

一般来说,皮肤肌肉丰厚的地方可稍深刺,如四肢踝腕关节以上,可针刺 0.2~0.3 寸。

Generally speaking, slightly deep needling can be performed on the part of skin with more muscle(such as the parts above ankle and wrist joints of four limbs), with the depth being 0.2-0.3 cun.

皮肤肌肉薄的地方浅刺,如头面部、井穴针刺深度常在 0.05 寸左右。

The shallow needling should be performed on the part of skin with less muscle(such as for the head, face and Jing-Well point), with the depth about 0.05 cun.

踝腕关节周围及以下、胸胁部穴位常控制在 0.1~0.2 寸。

The needling depth for the acupoints on the peripheral region of the ankle and wrist joints and the parts below them, and on the chest and hypochondrium is usually 0.1-0.2 cun.

泻时宜速刺,补时宜频频浅刺。

It is advisable to use rapid needling for reducing and repeated shallow needling for reinforcing.

年轻人、体质强壮者可稍深刺,老人、小孩宜浅刺,一般阿是穴、病变部位 要深刺 0.3~0.5 寸。

Slightly deep needling is applicable for young people and the person with strong constitution, and shallow needling is applicable for the elderly and children. Generally, deep needling should be performed on Ashi points and the lesion regions, with the depth being 0.3-0.5 cun.

针刺压痛点时,医者自觉手下沉紧感时应停止进针,针刺脓肿时针下出现 空虚感则止。

When doing acupuncture on tenderness points, the doctor should stop needling when feeling a burst of tension in the hand, and when inserting the needle in abscess, the doctor should stop needling when feeling void under the needle.

（三）施术后处理

（Ⅲ）Processing After Operation

1. **出针** 火针出针后,即用碘伏棉球或酒精棉球用力按压针孔,严禁揉按,以免出血,重而速按者可减轻或消除痛感。

1. Needle Withdrawal   After fire needle withdrawal, the acupuncture hole should be tightly pressed by iodophor or alcohol cotton balls. It is prohibited to knead the acupuncture hole, thereby avoiding bleeding. Pressing the acupuncture hole heavily and rapidly can relieve or eliminate painful sensation.

若火针针刺后出血,不必止血,待自然停止后用干棉球擦拭即可。

If bleeding occurs after fire needle therapy, there is no need to stop bleeding. Clean the acupuncture hole with dry cotton balls after bleeding stops naturally.

若以火针烙洞排脓或者割烙排脓者,务必使脓汁出尽,然后包扎,必要时宜加压包扎。

If use fire needle to cauterize hole to discharge pus or use cutting and cauterizing therapy to discharge pus, it is necessary to completely discharge pus and bind up. Use pressure dressing if necessary.

2. **疗程与间隔时间** 急性疾病每日或隔日 1 次,3 次为一疗程,慢性疾病 3~7 日 1 次,5~8 次为一疗程,两个疗程之间应该有 1~2 周的休息。

2. Course of Treatment and Interval Time   For acute diseases, the treatment is given every day or every other day with 3 times constituting one course; for the chronic diseases, the treatment is given every 3-7 days with 5-8 times constituting one course, and the interval between two courses is 1-2 weeks.

三、临床应用

Ⅲ. Clinical Application

（一）适应范围

（Ⅰ）Application Range

1. **外科** 化脓性皮脂腺囊肿、颈部淋巴结核、急性乳腺炎、乳腺增生症、乳腺纤维瘤、压疮、血栓闭塞性脉管炎、下肢静脉曲张、下肢慢性溃疡、丹毒、流行性腮腺炎等。

1. In Surgery   Suppurative sebaceous cyst, tuberculous lymphadenitis of

the neck, acute mastitis, hyperplasia of mammary glands, fibroadenoma of breast, pressure sore, thromboangitis obliterans, varix of lower limb, chronic ulcer of lower extremity, erysipelas, mumps, etc.

2. 骨科　颞下颌关节功能紊乱综合征、颈椎病、落枕、棘上韧带损伤、肌筋膜炎、腰椎间盘突出症、第三腰椎横突综合征、慢性腰肌劳损、腰肌扭伤、肩关节周围炎、肱骨外上髁炎、腕管综合征、关节扭伤、退行性膝关节炎、腘窝囊肿、跟痛症、腱鞘囊肿、慢性运动损伤、坐骨神经痛等。

2. In Orthopaedic　Temporomandibular joint disturbance syndrome, cervical spondylosis, stiff neck, damage of supraspinal ligament, myofascitis, prolapse of lumbar intervertebral disc, transverse process syndrome of third lumbar vertebra, chronic lumbar strain, lumbar muscle strain, periarthritis of shoulder, external humeral epicondylitis, carpal tunnel syndrome, joint sprain, degenerative knee arthritis, popliteal cyst, heel pain, ganglion cyst, chronic sports injury, sciatica, etc.

3. 内科　支气管炎、支气管哮喘、慢性胃炎、胃及十二指肠溃疡、慢性结肠炎、肠易激综合征、甲状腺功能减退、急性肾绞痛、失眠、偏头痛、慢性疲劳综合征、癔症性瘫痪、梅尼埃病、面神经炎、面肌痉挛、肋间神经痛、三叉神经痛、枕大神经痛、风湿性关节炎、强直性脊柱炎、类风湿关节炎、急性痛风性关节炎、癌症疼痛等。

3. In Internal Medicine　Bronchitis, bronchial asthma, chronic gastritis, gastroduodenal ulcer, chronic colitis, irritable bowel syndrome, hypothyroidism, acute renal colic, insomnia, migraine, chronic fatigue syndrome, hysterical paralysis, Ménière's disease, facial neuritis, facial spasm, intercostal neuralgia, trigeminal neuralgia, greater occipital neuralgia, rheumatic arthritis, ankylosing spondylitis, rheumatoid arthritis, acute gouty arthritis, cancer pain, etc.

4. 皮肤科　疣、湿疹、带状疱疹、白癜风、银屑病、神经性皮炎、瘙痒性皮肤病、虫咬皮炎、体表肿物、脂肪瘤、酒渣鼻、色素沉着、痤疮、冻疮等。

4. In Dermatology　Verruca, eczema, herpes zoster, vitiligo, psoriasis, neurodermatitis, itch of skin disease, insect dermatitis, goitre of body surface, lipoma, rosacea, hyperpigmentation, acne, frostbite, etc.

5. 妇科　痛经、月经不调、闭经、更年期综合征、慢性盆腔炎、子宫肌瘤、卵巢囊肿、不孕症等。

5. **In Gynecology** Dysmenorrhea, menstrual disorders, amenorrhoea, climacteric syndrome, chronic pelvic inflammatory disease, hysteromyoma, ovarian cyst, infertility, etc.

6. **男科** 前列腺炎、男子性功能障碍、不育症等。

6. **In Andrology** Prostatitis, male sexual dysfunction, sterility, etc.

7. **五官科** 睑腺炎、结膜炎、鼻炎、咽炎、牙痛、口腔溃疡等。

7. **In Ophthalmology and Otorhinolaryngology** Hordeolum, conjunctivitis, rhinitis, pharyngitis, toothache, oral ulcer, etc.

（二）**处方示例**

（Ⅱ）**Prescription Examples**

1. **郁证**

1. Depression Syndrome

（1）心脾两虚证、肝肾亏虚证：以细火针快速频频浅刺穴位 3~5 次，点刺深度 0.1~0.2 寸。

（1）Syndrome of deficiency of both heart and spleen, deficiency of liver and kidney: Repeatedly, quickly and shallowly insert thin fire needle into the acupoint for 3-5 times with the depth being 0.1-0.2 cun.

（2）肝气郁结证、痰气郁结证：以中粗火针，速刺法，点刺不留针，深度根据肌肉厚度而定，一般为 0.1~0.2 寸。

（2）Stagnation of liver qi, syndrome of phlegm-qi stagnation: Quickly insert medium thick fire needles into the acupoint, do point-pricking with no retaining of needle, and the insertion depth depends on muscle thickness, generally being 0.1-0.2 cun.

2. **带状疱疹** 阿是穴常规消毒，选用中粗火针于酒精灯上燃烧至发红后，采用围刺法，以刺穿疱疹、放出疱液为度。

2. **Herpes Zoster** After routine sterilization of Ashi points, the medium thick fire needles are taken to burn red by using alcohol burner, and encircling needling around the Ashi points is performed so as to pierce herpes and drain the follicular liquor out.

可配合拔火罐，留罐 5~10 分钟，起罐后用消毒棉球清除拔出的液体，再用

TDP 神灯照射 20 分钟。

The fire cupping therapy can be cooperatively used, the cup retaining time lasts for 5-10 minutes. Clean the drawn liquid with sterilized cotton ball after removing the cup, and then irradiate the acupoint with TDP Lamp for 20 minutes.

行间、太冲、侠溪、大都穴以细火针频频浅刺 3~5 次,点刺深度为 0.1~0.2 寸。余穴可采用快针法,深度根据肌肉厚度而定,一般为 0.1~0.2 寸。

Repeatedly and shallowly puncture Xingjian, Taichong, Xiaxi and Dadu points by using thin fire needles for 3-5 times, with point-needling depth being 0.1-0.2 cun; quick needling is conducted on remaining acupoints and the needling depth depends on muscle thickness, generally being 0.1-0.2 cun.

3. 腕管综合征 阿是穴常规消毒后,选用中粗火针于酒精灯上燃烧至通红后极快地刺入穴位,深度根据肌肉厚度而定,一般 0.1~0.2 寸,迅速出针,注意避开血管与神经。商阳、少商火针针刺深约 0.05 寸,余穴火针针刺深度 0.2~0.3 寸。

3. Carpal Tunnel Syndrome After routine sterilization of Ashi points, the medium thick fire needles are taken to burn very red by using alcohol burner. Very quickly insert the fire needles into Ashi points and the insertion depth depends on muscle thickness, usually being 0.1-0.2 cun. The needle should be rapidly withdrawn, and the operator should be careful to keep away from blood vessel and nerve. The fire needles on Shangyang and Shaoshang points should go about 0.05 cun in depth, and for the remaining acupoints, the depth is 0.2-0.3 cun.

(三)禁忌证

(Ⅲ) Contraindications

1. 高热、危重、糖尿病患者及孕妇慎用火针。

1. The fire needle therapy should be carefully used for the patients with hyperpyrexia, critical conditions, and diabetes as well as pregnant women.

2. 颜面、颈部和手足禁用火针。

2. It is prohibited on face, neck and hands and feet.

3. 疲劳过度、饥饿、过度紧张患者,不宜采用火针。

3. It is not applicable for the patients who feel over-fatigue, hunger and over-strain.

4. 火针针刺切忌刺入过深,避免损伤血管、肌腱、重要组织器官等。

4. Keep in mind that the fire needle should not be inserted too deep, avoiding damaging blood vessels, muscle tendon and important tissue and organ, etc.

(四) 注意事项
(Ⅳ) Precautions

1. 针前应充分同患者做好解释工作,避免患者紧张,患者以卧位为宜,减少晕针事件的发生。

1. Before treatment, explain the treatment fully to the patient to avoid patient's nervousness. It is appropriate for the patient to keep lying position to reduce fainting during acupuncture.

2. 注意用火安全,酒精灯不要灌得过满,一般占酒精灯容量的 2/3 以内为宜。

2. Pay attention to fire safety. The alcohol burner should not be overfilled, and it is advisable to make alcohol account for less than 2/3 of the capacity.

棉球蘸酒精不要过饱,防止烧伤患者皮肤、头发、汗毛等部位或衣物。

Cotton ball should not be dipped with too much alcohol, so to prevent the skin, hair, fine hair or other body parts of the patient and the clothing from burning.

3. 施用火针时应注意安全,防止火针灼伤患者其他部位或烧伤衣物。

3. When performing fire needle therapy, the operator should pay attention to fire safety, preventing other body parts of the patient or the clothing from burning.

4. 注意检查和维护针具,发现有剥蚀或缺损时,则不宜使用,以防意外。

4. Care should be taken to inspect and maintain the needling instrument, and if corroded or defected, the needling instrument would not be used to avoid accidents.

5. 针刺前要严格消毒施术局部皮肤,以 2%~5% 碘酒消毒后,再以 75% 酒精脱碘,消毒后在穴位局部涂上一层薄薄的跌打万花油,以防烫伤,减轻疼痛。

5. Before operation, the local skin should be first sterilized with 2%-5% iodine tincture , then given deiodination with 75% alcohol , and finally applied a thin layer of dieda wanhua oil to the acupoint, avoiding scald and alleviating pain.

6. 刺激量不宜过度,尤其对身体虚弱者。

6. The intensity of stimulus should not be too great, particularly for the patient with weak constitution.

7. 针柄及根处不要触及皮肤。

7. The needle handle and its root should not contact with skin.

8. 火针后一般不需要特殊处理,只需要用干棉球按压针孔即可。

8. No special treatment is needed generally after the fire needle operation, the acupuncture hole should be pressed with dry cotton balls.

如果用火针直接点刺创面,针刺后可按外科常规进行无菌处理。

In case that point needling is directly conducted on the wound surface, an aseptic processing should be given according to normal procedures of surgery.

如刺破血管而引起血流不止,可立即用消毒干棉球压迫止血。

If the blood vessels are pierced, resulting in continuous bleeding, hemostasis by compression should be immediately done with sterile dry cotton balls.

9. 接受火针治疗后,当天腧穴处皮肤可出现微红、灼热、轻度肿痛、痒等症状,属于正常现象,应嘱咐患者不必担心,不要用指甲搔抓,当日不要浸水,以防感染,忌食或少食辛辣之物,一般一周内会自行消失。

9. After fire needle treatment, skin at acupoint may be reddish, scorching, slightly swelling, and itching on the same day, which is a normal phenomenon. Instruct patient not to worry and not to scratch with nails. Prevent the skin from contacting with water on that day, avoiding infection. Avoid eating spicy food or eat less spicy food, and all the phenomena above will disappear automatically in general.

若红肿处出现脓点,要保持局部清洁,防止感染。

If red and swollen parts have pus points, the local skin should be kept clean for protecting from infection.

腧穴处红肿加重,分泌物增多,可外敷抗感染药膏等。

If red and swelling phenomenon at the acupoint becomes severe and secreta increases, anti-infective cream should be applied externally.

（五）意外的处理方法

（Ⅴ）Treatment for Accidents

1. **晕针** 发生针刺晕针现象,首先立即停止针刺,扶患者去枕平卧,头低脚高,松解衣带,同时注意保暖,可给患者喝温开水或糖开水,多可恢复。

1. Fainting During Acupuncture In case of fainting during acupuncture, firstly, immediately stop acupuncture, let patients lie in horizontal position (Trendelenburg position) with the clothing unloosed, and let the patients drink warm water or warm sugar water to keep them warm, which generally helps patients recover.

2. **断针** 安抚患者,消除紧张情绪,嘱咐患者保持原体位。

2. Breaking of Needle Reassure patients to eliminate their nervous mood and enjoin patients to keep original body position.

如皮肤尚露残端,可用镊子夹出。

If projecting from the surface of the skin, the needle stump should be taken out with tweezers.

若残端与皮肤相平,断面仍可见,可用左手拇指、示指在针旁按压,使之下陷,使残端露出皮肤,右手持镊子轻巧拔出。

If the needle stump is even with the skin and the transverse section is visible, press the skin around the needle with the thumb and index finger of the left hand, make the needle stump project from the surface of the skin and deftly draw the needle stump with tweezers held by right hand.

如残端没入皮内,需视所在部位,采用外科手术切开寻取。

If the needle stump is hidden in the skin, a surgical incision on the place where it is located should be performed to find it.

3. **出血** 如局部出现肿胀,应及时用棉球按压针孔周围 10 余分钟,不要揉动,其后可用 75% 酒精棉球轻压外敷,12 小时后肿胀部位可用热毛巾热敷,血脓已成,当时未散者,一般需 1~2 周方可吸收。

3. Bleeding For swelling in local skin, immediately press the skin around the acupuncture hole with cotton balls for about 10 minutes and do not knead. Next, lightly press and externally apply a compress by using the cotton balls with 75% alcohol, and 12 hours later, apply a hot compress to the swelling position

with hot towel. For a case with formed sanguinopurulent substances but with no diabrosis, complete absorption generally requires 1-2 weeks.

4. 针口疼痛　如已出现疼痛较重者,可快速用干棉球按压针孔,以减轻疼痛。

4. Pain in Acupuncture Hole　For the patient with severe pain, press the acupuncture hole with dry cotton balls quickly to relieve pain.

5. 针口感染　应结合症状,必要时外敷或口服使用抗感染药物。

5. Infection of Acupuncture Hole　Externally apply or take orally anti-infective drug according to the symptoms when necessary.

参 考 文 献
References

[1] 林国华,李丽霞.火针疗法[M].北京:中国医药科技出版社,2012.
[2] 尹远平,郝学君.中国特种针法临症全书[M].沈阳:辽宁科学技术出版社,2000.
[3] 王华,杜元灏.针灸学[M].北京:中国中医药出版社,2012.

第四节　耳　　针
Section 4　Auricular Acupuncture

耳针疗法为使用一定方法刺激耳穴以防治疾病的治疗方法。

Auricular acupuncture is a therapy in which certain methods are used to stimulate auricular acupoints for prevention and cure of diseases.

耳针疗法以中医学耳与经络、脏腑的内在联系为基础,结合全息理论与耳郭的表面解剖,在耳郭分区确定耳穴,治疗时遵循按相应部位选穴、按脏腑辨证选穴、按经络辨证选穴、按西医理论选穴、按临床经验选穴等原则进行耳穴选取,使用一定方法刺激耳穴,以预防与治疗全身疾病。

Based on the inner connection of ears with meridians, collaterals and zang-fu organs in TCM, auricular acupuncture therapy is combined with the holographic theory and the surface anatomy of auricles to determine the auricular acupoints in the auricular region. During treatment, principles such as acupoint selection according to the corresponding parts, acupoint selection according to syndrome differentiation of zang-fu organs, acupoint selection according to syndrome differentiation of meridians and collaterals, acupoint selection according to the western medicine theory, and acupointselection according to the clinical experience are followed to select the auricular acupoints, and then some methods are used to stimulate the auricular acupoints for prevention and cure of systemic diseases.

运用耳穴治疗疾病的历史很悠久,《灵枢·五邪》记载:"邪在肝,则两胁中痛……取耳间青脉以去其掣。"《灵枢·厥病》称:"耳聋无闻,取耳中。"唐代《备急千金要方》中有取耳穴治疗黄疸、寒暑疫毒等病的记载。

The use of auricular acupoints to treat diseases has a long history. According to the *Lingshu-Five Pathogens*: Pathogens in the liver will cause traction pain in the ribs, which can be removed by selecting blue veins in auricles. According to the *Lingshu-Jue Disease*: Ear center is selected for treatment of deafness. Selection of auricular acupoints for treatment of jaundice, cold and summer-heat, epidemic toxin, etc. is recorded in the *Essential Recipes for Emergent Use Worth A Thousand Gold* at Tang Dynasty.

后世文献常见用针、灸、熨、按摩、耳道塞药等方法刺激耳郭以防治疾病的记载,亦有以望、触耳郭的方法以诊断疾病的论述。

According to the later literatures, acupuncture, moxibustion, hot medicinal compress, massage, auditory canal suppositories and others are commonly used to stimulate auricles for prevention and cure of diseases, and inspection and touch of auricles are performed to diagnose diseases.

耳与经络联系密切。

Ears are closely connected with meridians and collaterals.

《阴阳十一脉灸经》记述了"耳脉",《内经》对耳与经络的关系做了较详细阐述,如《灵枢·口问》所言:"耳者,宗脉之所聚也。"手太阳、手足少阳、手阳明等经脉、经别都入耳中,足阳明、足太阳的经脉则分别上耳前、至耳上角。

Ear vessels are described in the *Moxibustion Canon of Eleven Vessels of Yin-yang System*, and the connection of ears with meridians and collaterals is elaborated in the *Inner Canon of Huangdi*. According to the *Lingshu-Oral*

Instruction：Ears are the parts where meridians converge. Hand-Taiyang, hand-foot-Shaoyang, hand-Yangming and other meridians, meridian divergencies converge in ears. The meridians of foot-Yangming and foot-Taiyang go to the preauricular region and run to the ear apex respectively.

六阴经虽不直接入耳,但都通过经别与阳经相合,而与耳相联系。

Six Yin meridians do not directly converge in ears, but they connect with their correlative Yang meridians through meridian divergencies, thus correlate with ears.

因此,十二经脉都直接或间接上达于耳。

Therefore, twelve meridians directly or indirectly go up to ears.

奇经八脉中阴跷、阳跷脉并入耳后,阳维脉循头入耳。

Yinqiao and Yangqiao of the eight extra meridians converge behind ears, and Yangwei meridian goes up to the head and then into ears.

耳与脏腑的生理功能、病理变化也密切相关。

The ears are closely related with the zang-fu organs physiologically and pathologically.

《内经》《难经》记载了耳与五脏之间生理功能上的联系。

The connection between ears and five zang organs in physiological function is recorded in the *Inner Canon of Huangdi* and the *Classic of Questioning*.

如《灵枢·脉度》言:"肾气通于耳,肾和则耳能闻五音矣。"《难经·四十难》说:"肺主声,故令耳闻声。"后世医家更为详细地论述了耳与脏腑的关系,如《证治准绳》说:"肾为耳窍之主,心为耳窍之客。"《厘正按摩要术》将耳郭分属五脏:"耳珠属肾,耳轮属脾,耳上轮属心,耳皮肉属肺,耳背玉楼属肝。"人体脏腑或躯体有病变时,往往在耳郭的相应部位出现压痛敏感、变形、变色和皮肤电阻特异性改变等反应,临床中可参考这些现象来诊断疾病,并通过刺激这些部位防治疾病。

According to the *Lingshu-Meridian Measurement*：Kidney qi connects with ears. As the kidney functions well, ears can hear five notes. According to the *Classic of Questioning-Problem 40*：The lung takes charge of voice, thus making ears hear voice. The physicians of later ages discuss the connection between ears and zang-fu organs in much more detail. According to the *Standards of Diagnosis and Treatment*: Nephrosis is the main cause for aural diseases, and cardiac abnormality is the secondary cause for aural diseases. In the *Revised Synopsis of Massage*, the auricle is divided into five parts respectively relating to five zang organs: The tragus belongs to the kidney, the helix to the spleen, the upper helix to the heart, the ear skin and flesh to the lung, and the ear back to the liver. When there are lesions in zang-fu organs or bodies, tenderness, deformation, color change, specific skin resistance changes and other reactions often appear in the corresponding parts of the auricle, and these phenomena can be clinically referenced to prevent and cure diseases by stimulating these regions.

为了便于交流和研究,中华人民共和国国家标准 GB/T 13734—2008《耳穴名称与定位》于 2008 年 7 月 1 日正式实施。

In order to facilitate communication and research, the PRC National Standard GB/T 13734-2008 *Auricular Name and Location* was formally implemented on July 1, 2008.

一、耳针刺激部位

I. Stimulating Parts of Auricular Acupuncture

将耳郭分为耳郭正面、耳郭背面和耳根 3 部分,耳穴分布其中,耳穴在耳郭的分布犹如一个倒置在子宫内的胎儿,其分布规律是:与面颊相应的穴位在耳垂,与上肢相应的穴位在耳舟,与躯干和下肢相应的穴位在对耳轮体部和对耳轮上、下脚,与内脏相应的穴位集中在耳甲。

The auricle is divided into three parts, that is, front, back and root, where auricular acupoints are distributed. Auricular acupoints are distributed in the auricle like an inverted fetus in the womb, which shows that the acupoints corresponding to the cheeks lie in the earlobes, those corresponding to the upper limbs in the scapha, those corresponding to the trunk and lower limbs in the principal part of antihelix, superior crura of antihelix and inferior crura of antihelix, and those corresponding to the viscera in the auricular concha.

耳穴定位示意图如下(图 1-5):

The diagram of auricular location is as follows (Fig. 1-5):

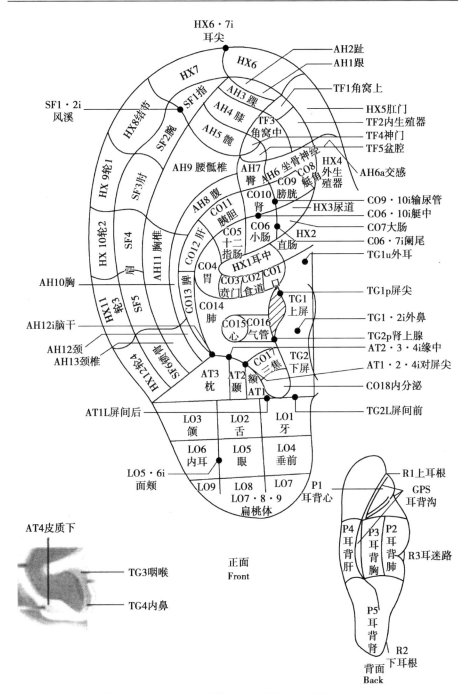

HX6·7i Ear Apex;SF1·2i Wind Stream;AH2 Toe;AH1 Heel;TF1 Superior Triangle Fossa;
HX5 Anus;TF2 Internal Genitals;TF4 Shenmen;TF5 Pelvis;AH6a Sympathetic;CO9·10i Ureter;
CO6·10i Center of Superior Concha;CO7 Large Intestine;CO6·7i Appendix;TG1u External Ear;

TG1·2i External Nose;TG2p Adrenal Gland;AT2·3·4i Central Rim;AT1·2·4i Apex of Antitragus;
AH10 Chest;AH12i Brain Stem;AH12 Neck;AH13 Cervical Vertebra;AT1L Posterior Intertragal
Notch;TG2L Anterior Intertragal Notch;LO5·6i Cheek;AT4 Subcortex;TG3 Pharynx and
Larynx;TG4 Internal Nose;R1 Upper Eardrum;P1 Heart of Posterior Surface;GPS Groove
of Posterior Surface;P4 Liver of Posterior Surface;P3 Chest of Posterior Surface;P2 Lung
of Posterior Surface;R3 Root of Ear Vagus;P5 Kidney of Posterior Surface;R2 Lower Ear
Root;HX9 Helix 1;HX10 Helix 2;HX11 Helix 3;HX12 Helix 4;HX8 Node;SF6 Clavicle;
SF4-SF5 Shoulder;SF3 Elbow;SF2 Chest;SF1 Finger;AH3 Ankle;AH4 Knee;
AH5 Hip;AH9 Lumbosacral Vertebrae;AH 11 Thoracic Vertebra;TF3 Middle Triangular Fossa;
AH8 Abdomen;AH7 Buttocks;AH6 Sciatic Nerve;HX4 External Genitals;CO13 Spleen;
CO12 Liver;CO11 Pancreas and Gallbladder;CO10 Kidney;CO9 Bladder;CO8 Angle
of Superior Concha;CO6 Small Intestine;CO5 Duodenum;CO4 Stomach;CO3 Cardia;
CO2 Esophagus;CO1 Mouth;CO14 Lung;HX3 Urethra;HX2 Rectum;HX1 Ear Center;
CO15 Heart;CO16 Trachea;TG1 Upper Tragus;TG2 Lower Tragus;CO17 Sanjiao;
AT3 Occiput;AT2 Temple;AT1 Forehead;LO3 Jaw;LO2 Tongue;LO1 Teeth;LO6 Internal
Ear;LO5 Eye;LO4 Anterior Ear Lobe;LO7-8-9 Tonsil.

图 1-5 耳穴定位示意图
Fig. 1-5 Diagram of auricular location

二、耳针操作技术

II. Operation Techniques of Auricular Acupuncture

(一) 操作前准备

(I) Preparation before Operation

1. **针具及压丸选择** 针具针身应光滑、无锈蚀,针尖应锐利、无倒钩,压丸应大小适宜、不易碎、无毒。

1. Selection of Needles and Ear Beans Needle body should be smooth without rust,the tip of needle should be sharp without barbs. The ear beans should be of the proper size,non-fragile and non-toxic.

2. **耳穴选择** 根据病情选择耳穴。

2. Selection of Auricular Acupoints Auricular acupoints should be selected according to the patient's condition.

3. **体位选择** 选择患者舒适,医者便于操作的治疗体位。

3. Position Selection The position selected should be comfortable for patients and easy for the doctor to operate.

4. **环境要求** 环境应清洁卫生,避免污染。

4. Environmental Requirements　The environment should be clean and hygienic and protected from contamination.

5. 消毒

5. Sterilization

（1）针具消毒：宜选择一次性针具。

（1）Needling instruments sterilization：It is advisable to select disposable needling instruments.

（2）部位消毒：应用含 75% 医用乙醇或 0.5%~1% 碘伏的棉签或棉球在施术部位擦拭。

（2）Site sterilization：The cotton swab or cotton ball with 75% medical ethanol or 0.5%-1% iodophor should be used at the operation sites.

（3）医者消毒：医者双手可先用肥皂水清洗干净，再用含 75% 医用乙醇或 0.5%~1% 碘伏棉球擦拭。

（3）Sterilization of doctor：The doctor should first wash hands with soapy water，and then brush hands with the cotton balls of 75% medical ethanol or 0.5%-1% iodophor to sterilize.

（二）施术方法

（Ⅱ）Operation Method

1. 耳穴毫针法　医者一手固定耳郭，另一手拇、食、中指持针刺入耳穴。

1. Auricular Filiform Needle Method　The doctor fixes the patient's auricle by one hand and holds the needle to puncture the auricular acupoints by the thumb，index finger and middle finger of the other hand.

针刺方向视耳穴所在部位灵活掌握，针刺深度宜 0.1~0.3cm，以不穿透对侧皮肤为度。

The needling direction should be flexibly controlled according to the sites where auricular acupoints are，and the needling depth should be 0.1-0.3cm，so as not to penetrate the opposite skin.

针刺手法与留针时间应视患者的病情、体质及耐受度综合考虑，宜留针 15~30 分钟，留针期间宜间断行针 1~2 次。

The needling techniques and the needle retaining time should be determined according to the patient's condition, constitution and tolerance. The needle should be retained for 15-30 minutes, and the manipulation of the needle should be performed 1-2 times during needle retention.

出针时一手固定耳郭,另一手将针拔出,应用无菌干棉球或棉签按压针孔。

During needle withdrawal, the auricle is fixed by one hand, and the needle is withdrawn by the other hand. The acupuncture hole should be pressed with a sterile dry cotton ball or cotton swab.

2. 耳穴压丸法 医者一手固定耳郭,另一手用镊子夹取耳穴压丸贴片贴压耳穴并适度按揉,根据病情嘱患者定时按揉。

2. Auricular-Plaster Therapy with Beans The operator fixes the patient's auricle by one hand and clamps the auricular plaster with tweezers by the other hand for auricular bean pressing with kneading manipulation performed moderately. According to the patient's condition, the patient should be asked to perform the regular kneading manipulation by oneself.

宜留置 2~4 天。

The auricular plaster should be retained for 2-4 days.

3. 耳穴埋针法 医者一手固定耳郭,另一手用镊子或止血钳夹住揿针针柄刺入耳穴,用医用胶布固定并适度按压,根据病情嘱患者定时按压。

3. Auricular Needle Embedding Therapy The operator fixes the patient's auricle by one hand and clamps the handle of thumb-tag needle with tweezers or hemostatic forceps to push the needle into the auricular acupoint, fix it with medical rubberized fabric, and then moderately perform pressing. According to the patient's condition, the patient should be asked to perform regular pressing by oneself.

宜留置 1~3 天后取出揿针,应消毒埋针部位。

The thumb-tag needle for subcutaneous embedding should be retained for 1-3 days, and the embedded needle site should be sterilized after the needle is withdrawn.

4. 耳穴刺血法 刺血前宜按摩耳郭使所刺部位充血。

4. Auricular Pricking Blood Therapy Massage should be performed on the sites of the auricle to be pricked before pricking.

医者一手固定耳郭,另一手持针点刺耳穴,挤压使之适量出血。

The doctor fixes the patient's auricle by one hand and holds the needle to perform quick puncture on the auricular acupoints by the other hand,squeezing it for a moderate amount of bleeding.

施术后用无菌棉球或棉签压迫止血并消毒刺血部位。

After operation,the pricking site should be stanched by compression and sterilized with a sterile cotton ball or a cotton swab.

5. 耳穴穴位注射法 是将微量药物注入耳穴的治疗方法。

5. Auricular Acupoint Injection It is a treatment method that a minute dose of medicine is injected into the auricular acupoints.

一般使用 1ml 注射器和 26 号注射针头,依病情选用相应的药物和耳穴。

1 ml syringe and No.26 syringe needle are generally used,and the corresponding medicine and auricular acupoints are selected according to the patient's condition.

操作时,左手固定耳郭,右手持注射器刺入已消毒的耳穴皮内或皮下,缓缓推入 0.1~0.3ml 药物,耳郭可有痛、胀、红、热等反应。

In operation,the doctor fixes the patient's auricle by the left hand,takes a syringe by the right hand and push it into the sterilized auricular acupoint intracutaneously or subcutaneously and then inserts 0.1-0.3ml medicine slowly. This operation may cause the auricle to have painful,swelling,blushing and burning reactions.

注射完毕后,用无菌干棉球轻轻按压针孔。

After injection,the acupuncture hole is gently pressed with a sterile cotton ball.

三、临床应用

III. Clinical Application

(一) 适应范围
(I) Application Range

1. 疼痛性疾病 如各种扭、挫伤等外伤性疼痛,头痛、肋间神经痛等神经性疼痛,手术后伤口痛及胃痛、胆绞痛等内脏痛等。

1. **Painful Diseases** Traumatic pain such as various sprains and contusions, neuropathic pain such as headache and intercostal nerve pain, postoperative wound pain, and visceral pain such as stomachache, biliary colic.

2. **炎性疾病及传染病** 如急慢性结肠炎、牙周炎、咽喉炎、扁桃体炎、胆囊炎、流行性感冒、百日咳、菌痢、腮腺炎等。

2. **Inflammatory Diseases and Infectious Diseases** Acute and chronic colitis, periodontitis, pharyngolaryngitis, tonsillitis, cholecystitis, influenza, pertussis, bacillary dysentery, parotitis, etc.

3. **功能紊乱性疾病** 如胃肠神经官能症、心脏神经官能症、心律不齐、高血压、眩晕症、多汗症、月经不调、遗尿、神经衰弱、癔症等。

3. **Dysfunctional Disorders** Gastrointestinal neurosis, cardiac neurosis, arrhythmia, hypertension, vertigo, hyperhidrosis, menstrual disorders, enuresis, neurasthenia, hysteria, etc.

4. **过敏及变态反应性疾病** 如荨麻疹、哮喘、变应性鼻炎、过敏性结肠炎、过敏性紫癜等。

4. **Allergy and Allergic Disorders** Urticaria, asthma, allergic rhinitis, allergic colitis, allergic purpura, etc.

5. **内分泌代谢紊乱性疾病** 如甲状腺功能亢进或减退、糖尿病、肥胖症、更年期综合征等。

5. **Endocrine and Metabolic Disorders** Hyperthyroidism or hypothyroidism, diabetes mellitus, obesity, climacteric syndrome, etc.

6. **其他** 耳针可用于催乳、催产,预防和治疗输血、输液反应,还可用于美容、戒烟、戒毒、延缓衰老、防病保健等。

6. **Others** Auricular acupuncture can be used to promote lactation, hasten parturition, prevent and treat blood transfusion reaction and injection reaction, and can also be used for beauty treatment, smoking cessation, drug withdrawal, anti-aging, disease prevention, health care, etc.

(二) 选穴原则

(Ⅱ) Acupoint Selection Principle

1. **按相应部位选穴** 选用与病变部位相对应的耳穴。

1. Selection of Acupoints According to Corresponding Sites   The auricular acupoints relevant to the lesion regions are selected.

如胃病取"胃"穴,痤疮取"面颊"穴等。

For example, stomach acupoints are selected for stomach disease, and cheek acupoints are selected for acnes.

2. **按脏腑辨证选穴**   根据脏腑理论,按各脏腑的生理功能和病理反应辨证取穴。

2. Selection of Acupoints According to Syndrome Differentiation of Zang-Fu Organs   The acupoints are selected according to syndrome differentiation based on the zang-fu organs theory, the physiological functions and pathological reactions of each organ.

如脱发取"肾"穴,皮肤病取"肺"穴、"大肠"穴等。

For example, kidney acupoints are selected for alopecia, and lung and large intestine acupoints are selected for dermatosis.

3. **按经络辨证选穴**   根据十二经脉循行和其病候取穴。

3. Selection of Acupoints According to Syndrome Differentiation of Meridians and Collaterals   The acupoints are selected according to the law of running course of the twelve meridians and their disease syndromes.

如坐骨神经痛,取"膀胱"穴或"胰胆"穴,牙痛取"大肠"穴等。

For example, bladder acupoints or pancreas and gallbladder acupoints are selected for sciatica, and large intestine acupoints are selected for toothache.

4. **按西医理论选穴**   耳穴中一些穴名是根据西医理论命名的,如交感、肾上腺、内分泌等。

4. Selection of Acupoints According to Western Medicine Theory   The names of some auricular acupoints are named according to the western medicine theory, such as sympathetic acupoint, adrenal gland acupoint, endocrine acupoint, etc.

这些穴位的功能基本与西医理论一致,选穴时应予以考虑。

The functions of these acupoints are basically consistent with the western medicine theory, which should be considered in acupoint selection.

如炎性疾病取"肾上腺"穴。

For example, adrenal gland acupoints are selected for inflammatory diseases.

5. 按临床经验选穴 临床实践发现有些耳穴具有治疗本部位以外疾病的作用,如"外生殖器"穴可以治疗腰腿痛。

5. Selection of Acupoints According to Clinical Experience It is found in clinical practice that some of the auricular acupoints have the effect of treating diseases besides their corresponding body parts. For example, the external genitals acupoints are selected for lumbago or leg pain.

(三)处方示例

(Ⅲ) Prescription Examples

1. 便秘 耳针法:选大肠、直肠、交感、皮质下。

1. Constipation Auricular acupuncture: Large intestine acupoint, rectum acupoint, sympathetic acupoint and subcortex acupoint are selected.

毫针刺,中等强度刺激或弱刺激,或使用耳穴压丸法、耳穴埋针法。

Filiform needles are used for puncture: Medium or weak intensity of stimulation is performed. Or auricular-plaster therapy with beans or auricular needle embedding therapy is used.

2. 眩晕

2. Vertigo

(1)肝阳上亢证

(1) Syndrome of Upper Hyperactivity of Liver Yang

主穴:肾上腺、皮质下、额。

Major Acupoints: Adrenal gland acupoint, subcortex acupoint and forehead acupoint.

配穴:肝、胆。

Supplement Acupoints: Liver acupoint and gallbladder acupoint.

(2)痰浊中阻证

(2) Syndrome of Phlegm-Turbidity Obstructing Middle Jiao

主穴:肾上腺、皮质下、额。

Major Acupoints：Adrenal gland acupoint，subcortex acupoint and forehead acupoint.

配穴：脾。

Supplement Acupoint：Spleen acupoint.

（3）气血亏虚证

（3）Syndrome of Deficiency of Both Qi and Blood

主穴：肾上腺、皮质下、额。

Major Acupoints：Adrenal gland acupoint，subcortex acupoint and forehead acupoint.

配穴：脾、胃。

Supplement Acupoints：Spleen acupoint and stomach acupoint.

（4）肾精不足证

（4）Syndrome of Insufficiency of Kidney Essence

主穴：肾上腺、皮质下、额。

Major Acupoints：Adrenal gland acupoint，subcortex acupoint and forehead acupoint.

配穴：肾、脑。

Supplement Acupoints：Kidney acupoint and brain acupoint.

上述耳针施术时，以毫针刺法或使用耳穴压丸法、耳穴埋针法。

During the above application of auricular acupuncture，filiform needle puncture is performed. Or auricular-plaster therapy with beans or auricular needle embedding therapy may be used.

3. 痛经　耳针法：选内生殖器、交感、皮质下、内分泌、神门、肝、肾、腹。

3. Dysmenorrhea　Auricular Acupuncture：Selection of internal genitals acupoint，sympathetic acupoint，subcortex acupoint，endocrine acupoint，shenmen acupoint，liver acupoint，kidney acupoint and abdomen acupoint are selected.

每次选取 2~4 穴，在所选取的穴位处寻找敏感点，快速捻转数分钟，每日或隔日 1 次，每次留针 20~30 分钟，或使用耳穴压丸法、耳穴埋针法。

Each time 2-4 acupoints may be selected and the sensitive points are searched at the selected acupoints. Quick twirling of needle is performed for a few minutes, once a day or every other day, with retention of needle lasting for 20-30 minutes. Or auricular-plaster therapy with beans or auricular needle embedding therapy may be used.

(四) 禁忌证
(Ⅳ) Contraindications

1. 局部脓肿、溃破、冻疮的耳穴禁用。

1. The auricular acupoints where there are partial abscess, diabrosis or chilblain are prohibited.

2. 凝血机制障碍患者禁用耳穴刺血法。

2. For patients suffering from dysfunction of blood coagulation, auricular pricking blood therapy is prohibited.

(五) 注意事项
(Ⅴ) Precautions

1. 施术部位应防止感染。

1. The operation sites should be protected from infection.

2. 紧张、疲劳、虚弱患者宜卧位针刺以防晕针。

2. The patients with tension, fatigue and weakness should be operated in the lying position to avoid fainting during acupuncture.

3. 湿热天气,耳穴压丸、耳穴埋针留置时间不宜过长,耳穴压丸宜 2~3 天,耳穴埋针宜 1~2 天。

3. For sticky weather, the retaining duration for auricular plaster therapy with beans and auricular needle embedding therapy should not be too long. For the former, it may last 2-3 days, and for the latter, 1-2 days.

4. 耳穴压丸、耳穴埋针留置期间应防止胶布脱落或污染。

4. During the retaining time in auricular plaster therapy with beans and auricular needle embedding therapy, the attention should be paid to protect the rubberized fabric from falling off or being contaminated.

对普通胶布过敏者宜改用脱敏胶布。

For the patients with allergy to the ordinary rubberized fabric, the desensitizing rubberized fabric can be used.

5. 耳穴刺血施术时,医者避免接触患者血液。

5. During the operation of auricular pricking blood therapy, the doctor should avoid touching the blood of the patient.

6. 妊娠期慎用耳针。

6. For women with pregnancy, auricular acupuncture should be used with caution.

参 考 文 献
References

[1] 石学敏. 针灸学[M]. 北京:中国中医药出版社,2002.

[2] 中国针灸学会. 针灸技术操作规范 第3部分:耳针:GB/T 21709.3—2008[S]. 北京:中国标准出版社,2010.

[3] 王华,杜元灏. 针灸学[M]. 北京:中国中医药出版社,2012.

第五节 过 梁 针
Section 5 Penetration Needle

过梁针由古代"九针"中的"长针""大针"发展演变而来,是一种长而粗大的针具。

Penetration needle is developed and evolved from "long needle" and "big needle" in ancient "nine forms of needles". It is a long and thick needle.

过梁针法是针刺的一种透穴法,其雏形源于《灵枢·官针》记载的合谷刺、恢刺等刺法,又称深刺奇穴法。

Penetration needle therapy is an acupoint penetration method and its prototype originates from acupuncture techniques such as Hegu needling and restoration needling recorded in the *Lingshu-Guanzhen*, also called as deep puncture at extra points.

以毫针深刺或强刺激经外奇穴,以不穿透对侧皮肤为度,具有针体粗、针身长、取穴少、进针深、刺激量强、见效快的特点。

It executes deep puncture with filiform needle or strongly stimulates the extra points to the degree of not piercing the opposite skin. It has the features of thick needle body, long needle body, selection of fewer acupoints, deep needling, strong quantity of stimulus and quick effects.

《灵枢·九针论》曰:"长针,取法于綦针,长七寸,主取深邪远痹者也。"又有"八正之虚风,八风伤人,内舍于骨解腰脊节腠理之间,为深痹也,故为之治针,必长其身,锋其末"之说。

It is said in the *Lingshu-Jiuzhen Lun* that long needles are sharp and thin, have a length of 7 cun and are used to treat obstinate arthralgia with strong invasion of pathogens. If wind pathogen invades the human body and goes deep into human bony suture, lumbar spinal joints and striae and interstitial space, it will cause obstinate diseases. In order to treat the diseases, long needles are made, and the needles should have a longer body and a sharper point.

《灵枢·官针》曰:"病在中者,取以长针。"指出长针适宜于治疗深邪远痹和病在内部深层之痼疾。

It is said in the *Lingshu-Guanzhen* that internal disease should be treated by long needles. It indicates that the long needle is suitable for treating obstinate arthralgia with strong invasion of pathogens as well as intractable diseases in internal deep parts of the body.

过梁针疗法在古籍中无专门论述,流传于民间,主要治疗精神、神经科疾病,对癔症性瘫痪、精神分裂症、癫、狂、痫等疾病疗效尤为显著。

Penetration needle therapy is not specially discussed in ancient books. It is widely spread among the people, mainly treats mental diseases and neurological diseases and has notable curative effects on hysterical paralysis, schizophrenia, depressive psychosis, mania, epilepsy, etc.

一、选穴原则

I. Acupoint Selection Principle

过梁针是针刺的一种透穴法,选穴有"过梁针常用奇穴"与"经穴透穴"两部分。

Penetration needle therapy is an acupoint penetration method in needling，and its acupoint selection includes "common extra points of penetration needle" and "acupoint penetration".

过梁针常用特定奇穴,用穴少而精,有较明显的规律性,从部位上来看,多为关节、骨骼附近的腧穴,针刺深并透过肢体,一般是将针由肢体一侧透刺到肢体对侧皮下,以达到疗效。

Special extra points are frequently used in penetration needle therapy，the acupoints selected are fewer but better and have obvious regularity. From the view of positions，their locations are near joints and skeletons. The operation is a deep needling；generally，the needle is pierced from one side of the limbs to the opposite subcutaneous side of the limbs to achieve the curative effect.

经穴透穴,多选用与疾病相关的,位于肘膝肩关节或任督二脉等阴阳两条经脉的体位相对称的两个穴位为组穴,进行透刺得气,调整阴阳,治疗疾病。

For acupoint penetration，two symmetrical acupoints related to the disease and located in two yin-yang meridians of elbow，knee and shoulder joints or Ren and Du meridians are commonly selected as group acupoints to penetrate for getting the qi of acupuncture，regulating yin and yang and treating diseases.

应用过梁针,应根据病情,辨证施治,各穴所主治病症不同,针法亦各有不同,应根据病症,灵活应用。

Penetration needle therapy should be conducted according to treatment based on differentiation of symptoms and signs of the patient. Indications of diseases of each acupoint are different，and acupuncture manipulations are also different. Penetration needle therapy should be flexibly applied according to the diseases.

（一）过梁针常用奇穴

（Ⅰ）Common Extra Points of Penetration Needle

1. 天灵　定位:腋窝前缘直上 1 寸,向内旁开 5 分,垂膊取之。

1. Tianling　Locating：1 cun directly above anterior border of the axillary fossa，5 fen（a Chinese unit of length，1 fen equals 1/3 centimeter）laterally inwards. To locate the acupoint，let the patient hang the arm downwards naturally.

针法:进针时由腋窝前缘向外上方斜刺 1.5 寸,若病重,采用透刺法,刺入

5~6 寸。

Acupuncture operation：Obliquely puncture the acupoint from anterior and superolateral border of the axillary fossa with the tip of needle directly, in depth of 1.5 cun; and for serious diseases, the acupoint penetration needle therapy is performed, in depth of 5-6 cun.

主治：狂证，伤人自伤，口中唱骂，癫证，上肢瘫痪。

Indications：Mania, injuring others, self-injuring, cursing, depressive psychosis, and paralysis of the upper limbs.

2. 屈委阳 定位：屈肘，肘横纹端外 0.5 寸处。

2. Quweiyang Locating：0.5 cun laterally to the external end of the cubital crease as the elbow is flexed.

针法：进针时直刺 1.5 寸，若病重，由肘横纹外侧端向肘横纹内侧端透刺 2~3 寸。

Acupuncture operation：Vertically puncture in depth of 1.5 cun; and for serious diseases, puncture 2-3 cun from the lateral end of the cubital crease to the medial end of the cubital crease.

主治：躁动不安，精神分裂症，上肢瘫痪、僵直、颤抖。

Indications：Restlessness, schizophrenia, and paralysis, rigor, jitter of the upper limbs.

3. 尺桡 定位：前臂前区两筋间，腕横纹至肘横纹之中央，腕上 6 寸。

3. Radius Locating：Between two tendons of flexural aspect of the forearm at the middle way between the transverse crease of the wrist to the cubital crease, 6 cun above the wrist.

针法：进针时直刺 1.5 寸，若病重，由前臂前区端向前臂后区端透刺 2~3 寸。

Acupuncture operation：Vertically puncture in depth of 1.5 cun; and for serious diseases, puncture 2-3 cun from the flexural aspect of the forearm to the extensor aspect of the forearm.

主治：妄想型精神分裂症，郁证，焦虑症，上肢麻木、瘫痪、痉挛。

Indications：Paranoid schizophrenia, melancholia, anxiety disorders, and numbness, paralysis and spasm of upper limbs.

4. **中桡** 定位:前臂前区两筋间,腕横纹上 4 寸。

4. **Zhongrao** Locating:Between two tendons of flexural aspect of the forearm,4 cun above the transverse crease of the wrist.

针法:进针时直刺 1 寸,若病重,由前臂前区端向前臂后区端透刺 1.5~2.5 寸。

Acupuncture operation:Vertically puncture,by 1 cun in depth;and for serious diseases,puncture from flexural aspect of the forearm to extensor aspect of the forearm,1.5-2.5 cun in depth.

主治:轻度精神分裂症,癫证,上肢麻木、瘫痪、痉挛。

Indications:Light schizophrenia,depressive psychosis,and numbness, paralysis and spasm of upper limbs.

5. **寸桡** 定位:前臂前区两筋间,腕横纹上 2 寸(内关穴)。

5. **Cunrao** Locating:Between two tendons of flexural aspect of the forearm,2 cun above the transverse crease of the wrist(Neiguan point).

针法:进针时直刺 1 寸,若病重,由前臂前区端向前臂后区端透刺 1.5~2 寸。

Acupuncture operation:Vertically puncture,1 cun in depth;and for serious diseases,puncture the flexural aspect of the forearm to extensor aspect of the forearm,1.5-2 cun in depth.

主治:精神分裂症,癫证,上肢僵直,颤证。

Indications:Schizophrenia,depressive psychosis,rigidity of upper limbs,and tremor.

6. **虎边** 定位:在手背侧第 1、2 掌骨间,第 2 掌骨桡侧缘中点处。

6. **Hubian** Locating:Between the first and the second metacarpal bones in dorsal side,in the midpoint of the radial aspect of the second metacarpal bone.

针法:进针时直刺 0.5~1 寸,若病重,由掌背向掌心透刺 1~1.5 寸,刺时手呈半握拳状。

Acupuncture operation:Vertically puncture,0.5-1 cun in depth;and for serious diseases,puncture 1-1.5 cun from the dorsal side to the palmar side with the hand in half-closed fist shape during operation.

主治:带有持久激动症状的精神分裂症、狂证和其他带有激动症状的精神病。

Indications：Schizophrenia with persistent agitation symptom，mania and other psychosis with agitation symptom.

7. 阴委一　定位：仰卧屈膝，股外侧、腘横纹上 1 寸，股二头肌腱与股外侧肌凹陷处。

7. Yinwei Ⅰ　Locating：Lie in supine position with flexion of knees，at the lateral femur，1 cun above popliteal crease，and in the depression of tendon biceps femoris and musculus vastus lateralis.

针法：进针时直刺 3~4 寸，若病重，由股外侧向股内侧透刺 5~8 寸。

Acupuncture operation：Vertically puncture by 3-4 cun in depth；and for serious diseases，puncture 5-8 cun in depth，from the lateral femur to the medial femur.

主治：狂证，癫证，癔病，下肢瘫痪。

Indications：Mania，depressive psychosis，hysteria and paralysis of the lower limbs.

8. 阴委二　定位：仰卧屈膝，股外侧、腘横纹上 2 寸，股二头肌腱与股外侧肌凹陷处，阴委一向上 1 寸。

8. Yinwei Ⅱ　Locating：Lie in supine position with flexion of knees，at the lateral femur，2 cun above popliteal crease，in the depression of tendon biceps femoris and musculus vastus lateralis，and 1 cun above Yinwei Ⅰ.

针法：进针时直刺 3~4 寸，若病重，由股外侧向股内侧透刺 6~8 寸。

Acupuncture operation：Vertically puncture，3-4 cun in depth；and for serious diseases，puncture 6-8 cun in depth，from the lateral femur to the medial femur.

主治：狂证，精神分裂症，癫证，下肢瘫痪。

Indications：Mania，schizophrenia，depressive psychosis，and paralysis of the lower limbs.

9. 阴委三　定位：仰卧屈膝，股外侧、腘横纹上 3 寸，股二头肌腱与股外侧肌凹陷处，阴委二向上 1 寸。

9. Yinwei Ⅲ　Locating：Lie in supine position with flexion of knees，at the lateral femur，3 cun above popliteal crease，in the depression of tendon biceps femoris and musculus vastus lateralis, and 1 cun above Yinwei Ⅱ.

针法:进针时直刺 3~5 寸,若病重,由股外侧向股内侧透刺 7~8 寸。

Acupuncture operation: Vertically puncture, 3-5 cun in depth; and for serious diseases, puncture 7-8 cun in depth, from the lateral femur to the medial femur.

主治:精神分裂症,狂证,癫证,下肢瘫痪。

Indications: Schizophrenia, mania, depressive psychosis, and paralysis of the lower limbs.

10. 中平　定位:外膝眼下 5 寸,胫骨旁开 2 寸。

10. Zhongping　Locating: 5 cun under Waiqiyan, and 2 cun laterally away from the tibia.

针法:进针时由股外侧向内上方斜刺 3 寸,若病重,采用透刺法,刺入 4~6 寸。

Acupuncture operation: Obliquely puncture, 3 cun in depth, from the lateral femur to the supero-medial aspect; and for serious diseases, puncture 4-6 cun in depth by using an acupoint penetration needle therapy.

主治:精神病,精神分裂症,心因性反应症,癔病和神经官能症,下肢瘫痪、冷痛、麻木。

Indications: Psychosis, schizophrenia, psychogenic reaction, hysteria, neurosis, and paralysis, crymodynia, numbness of the lower limbs.

11. 灵宝　定位:股外侧,腘横纹上 6 寸,股外侧肌与股二头肌之间,阴委三上 3 寸。

11. Lingbao　Locating: In the lateral femur, 6 cun above popliteal crease, between the musculus vastus lateralis and the musculus biceps femoris, and 3 cun above Yinwei Ⅲ.

针法:进针时直刺 3~4 寸,若病重,由股外侧向股内侧透刺 7~8 寸。

Acupuncture operation: Vertically puncture, 3-4 cun in depth; and for serious diseases, puncture 7-8 cun in depth, from the lateral femur to the medial femur.

主治:带有持久激动症状的精神分裂症,狂证,癫证,下肢瘫痪。

Indications: Schizophrenia with persistent agitation symptom, mania, depressive psychosis, and paralysis of the lower limbs.

12. 脑根 定位：外踝与跟腱之间凹陷上 1 寸处（昆仑穴）。

12. Naogen Locating：1 cun above the depression between the lateral malleolus and the heel tendon（Kunlun point）.

针法：进针时直刺 1 寸，若病重，由外踝端向内踝端透刺 1.5~2.5 寸。

Acupuncture operation：Vertically puncture, 1 cun in depth；and for serious diseases, puncture 1.5-2.5 cun in depth, from the lateral malleolus aspect to the medial malleolus aspect.

主治：慢性精神病，精神分裂症恢复期，呆证，下肢痿软，肩背拘急疼痛。

Indications：Chronic psychosis, convalescence of schizophrenia, dementia, flaccidity of lower limbs, and acute pain in the shoulder and the back.

13. 立命 定位：人中穴旁开 1 寸。

13. Liming Locating：1 cun laterally away from philtrum.

针法：进针时由人中旁一侧向对侧平刺 1 寸，若病重，采用透刺法，刺入 1.5~2 寸。

Acupuncture operation：Horizontally puncture 1 cun, from the philtrum to the opposite side；and for serious diseases, puncture 1.5-2 cun by using acupoint penetration needle therapy.

主治：急、重型精神分裂症，狂证，郁证，癔病等。

Indications：Acute and serious schizophrenia, mania, melancholia, hysteria, etc.

14. 颈七 定位：在第七颈椎棘突隆起中。

14. Jingqi Locating：In the bulge of the seventh cervical spine.

针法：进针由颈后侧向内上侧斜刺 2~3 寸，若病重，采用透刺法，刺入 4~5 寸。

Acupuncture operation：Obliquely puncture 2-3 cun, from the posterior neck to the supero-medial aspect；and for serious diseases, puncture 4-5 cun by using acupoint penetration needle therapy.

主治：有激动症状的精神分裂症、狂证和较重的神经官能症等。

Indications：Schizophrenia with agitation symptom, mania, serious neurosis with emotional state, etc.

15. 胸七　定位：第七胸椎棘突高点处。

15. Xiongqi　Locating：In the bulge of the seventh thoracic spinous process.

针法：进针时由胸后侧向内上侧斜刺 2~3 寸，若病重，采用透刺法，刺入 4~5 寸。

Acupuncture operation：Obliquely puncture 2-3 cun，from the posterior chest to the supero-medial aspect；and for serious diseases，puncture 4-5 cun by using acupoint penetration needle therapy.

主治：无激动症状的精神分裂症，郁证，其他无激动兴奋状态的精神病及神经官能症等。

Indications：Schizophrenia without agitation symptom，melancholia and other psychosis and neurosis without emotional state，etc.

（二）经穴透穴常用腧穴

（Ⅱ）Common Acupoints of Acupoint Penetration

1. 神聪透神聪（由前向后透刺）　定位：百会穴前、后相去各 1 寸。

1. Penetrating through Shencong to Shencong（Acupoint Penetration）Locating：1 cun respectively anterior and posterior to Baihui point.

主治：各型精神分裂症，狂证，郁证，神经官能症等。

Indications：Various schizophrenia，mania，melancholia，neurosis，etc.

2. 神庭透前顶　定位：神庭在头部中线入发际 0.5 寸处。前顶在头部中线入前发际 3.5 寸处。

2. Penetrating through Shenting to Qianding　Locating：Shenting is on the midsagittal line of the head，0.5 cun within the anterior hairline. Qianding is on the midsagittal line of the head，3.5 cun within the anterior hairline.

主治：各型精神分裂症，狂证，郁证，神经官能症等。

Indications：Various schizophrenia，mania，melancholia，neurosis，etc.

3. 风池透风池　定位：在胸锁乳突肌与斜方肌上端之间凹陷中，平风府穴处。

3. Penetrating through Fengchi to Fengchi　Locating：In the depression between the upper portion of musculus sternocleidomastoid and musculus trapezius，and level with Fengfu point.

主治：精神疾病的好转恢复期。

Indications：Convalescence of mental diseases.

4. 太阳透率谷 定位：太阳穴在眉梢与目外眦连线中点外开 1 寸处的凹陷中。率谷穴在耳尖直上，入发际 1.5 寸处。

4. Penetrating through Taiyan to Shuaigu Locating：Taiyan is in the depression 1 cun posterior to the midpoint between the lateral end of the eyebrow and outer canthus. Shuaigu is superior to the auricular apex, 1.5 cun within the hairline.

主治：有持久激动症状的精神分裂症，狂证。

Indications：Schizophrenia with persistent agitation symptom and mania.

5. 膻中透华盖 定位：膻中穴在胸骨中线上，两乳头之间。华盖穴在前正中线上胸骨角的中点。

5. Penetrating through Danzhong to Huagai Locating：Danzhong is between the two mammillae on the midsternal line. Huagai is at the midpoint of the sternal angle on the anterior midline.

主治：无激动症状的精神分裂症，郁证，精神病和神经官能症等。

Indications：Schizophrenia without agitation symptom, melancholia, psychosis, neurosis, etc.

6. 巨阙透神阙 定位：巨阙在腹中线上，脐上 6 寸处。神阙，在脐窝中点处。

6. Penetrating through Juque to Shenque Locating：Juque is 6 cun above the navel on the midline of the abdomen. Shenque is at the center of navel.

主治：无激动症状的精神分裂症，郁证，精神病和神经官能症等。

Indications：Schizophrenia without agitation symptom, melancholia, psychosis, neurosis, etc.

7. 太冲透涌泉 定位：太冲在足背第 1、2 跖骨结合部之前凹陷中。涌泉在足掌（去趾）前 1/3 与后 2/3 交界之凹陷中。

7. Penetrating through Taichong to Yongquan Locating：Taichong is in the dorsal depression in front of the junction of 1st and 2nd metatarsal bones. Yongquan is in the palmar depression of the junction of anterior one third and two

thirds of the sole (excluding toes).

主治：有持久激动症状的精神分裂症，狂证。

Indications: Schizophrenia with persistent agitation symptom, and mania.

二、操作技术

Ⅱ. Operation Techniques

（一）操作前准备
（Ⅰ）Preparation Before Operation

1. **针具选择**　一般选用 22 号、20 号、18 号的 3 寸、6 寸、8 寸、1 尺的不锈钢毫针。

1. Selection of Needles　3cun, 6cun, 8cun and 1chi (a Chinese unit of length equals 1/3 meter) stainless steel filiform needles of No. 22, No. 20 and No. 18 are selected generally.

所选择的过梁针针身应光滑、无锈蚀，针尖应锐利、无倒钩。

Needle bodies of the selected penetration needles should be smooth without rust, and the tips of the needles should be sharp without barbs.

2. **体位选择**　选择患者舒适，医者便于操作的治疗体位。

2. Position Selection　The position selected should be comfortable for patients and easy for the doctor to operate.

3. **环境要求**　环境应清洁卫生，避免污染。

3. Environmental Requirements　The environment should be clean and hygienic and protected from contamination.

4. **消毒**　包括针具消毒、针刺部位消毒、医者消毒。

4. Sterilization　Including sterilization of needle, sterilization of acupuncture positions and sterilization of doctors.

（二）施术方法
（Ⅱ）Operation Method

1. **行针手法**　一般情况下多采用捻转、提插手法，如果需要强刺激或针感不明显时，可配合以刮法、摇法、循法、弹法、震颤法等稍重手法。

1. **Needling Manipulation**　Twirling of needle and lifting and thrusting of needle are frequently used generally. If strong stimulation is needed or needling sensation is not obvious, such heavier manipulations as scraping, shaking, touching along meridian, shaking maneuver, and vibration can be used in combination.

部分过梁针奇穴,须在针刺时出现感应,方能获效。

Some extra points of penetration needle therapy can effect only when there is a response during acupuncture.

如针刺阴委一等穴治疗癔症性瘫痪、外伤性截瘫、脱髓鞘疾病等,必须出现肢体不自主抽动或颤动,疗效才显著。

For example, acupuncture on Yinwei I, etc. to treat hysterical paralysis, traumatic paraplegia, demyelinating disease and other diseases can effect only when the limbs twitch or quiver spontaneously.

在过梁针后,部分病人会出现轻度头昏、微汗、乏力等针刺反应,有些精神分裂症和癔病患者,在出现这样的应激性反应后,可能会霍然而愈。

After penetration needle therapy, some patients may have acupuncture reactions such as light dizziness, slight sweating, lacking in strength, etc. Some patients with schizophrenia and hysteria may be instantly cheerful and cured after these irritable reactions occur.

应用过梁针,必须根据病情,辨证施治。

The penetration needle therapy must be applied according to patient's conditions to determine the treatment based on symptom differentiation.

奇穴主治病症不同,过梁针法亦各有所异。

Indications of extra points are different, so penetration needle methods are also different.

临证时,须根据治疗需要,灵活运用。

In clinical practice, penetration needle therapy should be flexibly used according to needs of treatment.

(1) 双手进针法:刺手拇指、示指、中指三指持针疾速直刺进皮,到达皮下后,左手夹持压倒针具,固定针孔处皮肤,右手小弧度捻转,缓慢进针。

(1) Needle insertion with both hands: With the thumb, forefinger and middle

finger of the needling hand, take the needle and quickly insert it into the skin. After the needle reaches the subcutaneous issue, the pressing hand holds and pushes down the needle to fix the skin at the acupuncture hole. The needling hand twirls the needle with a small radian and slowly inserts the needle.

进针到穴位深度的一半时，左手扶托于穴位肢体的对侧，以探测针尖到达的位置，直到进针至对侧皮下。

When the needle tip goes into half of the depth of the acupoints, the pressing hand supports the opposite side of the acupoint to detect the position where the needle tip reaches, and the needling hand inserts the needle further to the subcutaneous tissue on the opposite side.

针刺期间可配合开阖补泻、徐疾补泻、烧山火、透天凉等手法。

In acupuncture, such manipulations as open-close reinforcing-reducing, slow-rapid reinforcing-reducing, heat-producing and cold-inducing can be used in combination.

（2）静置留针法：留针期间不施行任何针刺手法，让针体留置在穴位内。

（2）Static retention of needle: Do not conduct any acupuncture technique during retention of needle, and let the needle body retain in the acupoint.

一般情况下，留针时间宜在 15~30 分钟，也可根据患者情况，适当延长或缩短留针时间。

Generally, the retention time of needle should be 15-30 minutes, and can also be appropriately prolonged or shortened according to the conditions of patients.

（3）过梁针补法：行"凤凰理羽"。

（3）Reinforcing method in penetration needle therapy: "Phoenix combs feather".

即拇指向前、食指向后捻转手法九次，三九二十七次，或九九八十一次。

That is, twirl the needle with the thumb forward and with the forefinger backward for 9 times, totally 27 times or 81 times.

留针期间，可间歇重复施行，每次 0.5~1 分钟。

In retention of needle, this manipulation can be done intermittently and repeatedly, 0.5-1 minutes each time.

（4）过梁针泻法：行"凤凰展翅"。

（4）Reducing method in penetration needle therapy："Phoenix spreads the wings".

即拇指向后、食指向前捻转手法六次，六六三十六次，或八八六十四次。

That is, twirl the needle with the thumb backward and with the forefinger forward for 6 times, totally 36 times or 64 times.

留针期间，可间歇重复施行，每次 0.5~1 分钟。

In retention of needle, this manipulation can be conducted intermittently and repeatedly, 0.5-1 minutes each time.

2. 出针要求　出针时手法宜轻，可采用与进针手法相似的手法，左手夹持针具，右手小弧度捻转，缓慢出针。

2. Requirements for Needle Withdrawal　In needle withdrawal, the action should be gentle. A technique similar to a needling technique can be adopted. The left hand holds the needle, and the right hand twirls the needle with small radian to slowly withdraw it.

出针后可适当休息 20 分钟，以便观察有无不适，方便及时处理。

After needle withdrawal, the patient may have an appropriate rest for 20 minutes so as to observe whether there is any discomfort, which facilitates the treatment in time.

3. 过梁针技术治疗间隔及疗程　一般情况下，是每日或隔日一次，10 天为一个疗程。

3. Treatment Interval and Course of Penetration Needle Therapy　Generally, once a day or once every other day; 10 days makes one course.

三、临床应用

Ⅲ. Clinical Application

（一）适应范围

（Ⅰ）Application Range

1. 精神性疾病　精神分裂症、狂证、郁证、焦虑症、神经官能症、更年期综合征、癔病。

1. In Psychiosis　Schizophrenia, mania, depression, anxiety, neurosis, climacteric syndrome and hysteria.

2. **神经内科**　面瘫、失眠、癫痫、偏瘫、神经麻痹。

2. In Neurology　Facial paralysis, insomnia, epilepsy, hemiplegia and nerve palsy.

3. **骨伤科**　肩周炎、腰痛、关节疼痛。

3. In Osteology and Traumatology　Scapulohumeral periarthritis, lumbago and arthralgia.

4. **外科**　胆囊炎、胆结石、肾积水、输尿管结石、膀胱结石。

4. In Surgery　Cholecystitis, cholelithiasis, hydronephrosis, ureteral calculus and bladder stone.

(二) 处方示例

(Ⅱ) Prescription Examples

1. **狂证**　常用穴位：阴委一、阴委二、阴委三、灵宝、屈委阳、天灵。

1. Mania　Frequently-Used Acupoints: Yinwei Ⅰ, Yinwei Ⅱ, Yinwei Ⅲ, Lingbao, Quweiyang and Tianling.

操作：若患者体格健壮，躁动有力，脉为实象，可给予重泻的手法。

Operation: If the patients are robust, restless and strong and have excess pulse, a heavy reducing technique can be given.

若患者有无力、冷汗、面色变白、脉搏频细、血压轻度下降等症状，这时应停止针刺，首先将上肢部针退出，让患者休息片刻，待其稍恢复后，再令患者大量喝水，并服中药散剂促使患者呕吐，吐止后再服泻剂，如患者不能自服可用鼻饲。

If the patients have the symptoms of weakness, cold sweat, pale complexion, rapid and thread pulse, slight decrease in blood pressure, etc. Immediately stop needling, withdraw the needle from the upper limbs and let the patients have a rest. After the patients slightly recover, let the patients to drink a great amount of water and take Chinese Materia Medicia (CMM) powder to enable the patients to vomit. After vomiting, let the patients take purgative medicine. If the patients cannot take the medicine by themselves, nasal feeding can be adopted.

像这样的针刺一般经过 1~3 次,患者躁动停止,表现合作(但药物的配合仅限于第一次),以后继续给以针刺,直至痊愈。(每次用的穴位渐次减少,手法也转用轻泻。若虽为狂证而脉象虚者,则需用"平补平泻"。)

After 1-3 times of such acupuncture, the patients may stop restlessness and gradually cooperate (but medical cooperation is only limited to the first time). Then, acupuncture is given until the patients are cured. (acupoints used each time are gradually reduced, and the technique changes to light reducing. If the patients have mania but have feeble pulse, "even reinforcing and reducing" should be used.)

2. **癫证** 常用穴位:阴委一、阴委二、阴委三、中平、脑根。

2. **Depressive Psychosis** Frequently-Used Acupoints: Yinwei Ⅰ, Yinwei Ⅱ, Yinwei Ⅲ, Zhongping and Naogen.

操作:此类患者多采用"多补少泻"手法,当患者表现合作后,则浅刺轻刺(不捻转)。

Operation: A "more-reinforcing and less-reducing" technique is often adopted for such patients. After the patients cooperate, shallow and light puncture (no twirling of needle) is conducted.

3. **痫证** 常用穴位:立命、阴委一、阴委二、阴委三,配以腰奇透腰阳关、大椎透神道、鸠尾透中脘、百会透神庭、膻中透鸠尾、心俞透胆俞。

3. **Epilepsy** Frequently-Used Acupoints: Liming, Yinwei Ⅰ, Yinwei Ⅱ and Yinwei Ⅲ, in combination with the penetrating through Yaoqi to Yaoyangguan, penetrating through Dazhui to Shendao, penetrating through Jiuwei to Zhongwan, penetrating through Baihui to Shenting, penetrating through Danzhong to Jiuwei and penetrating through Xinshu to Danshu.

操作:此类患者多采用"泻法",先予立命以强刺激,直至眼球湿润或流泪,若患者已见好转,则用其他上述穴位进行治疗。

Operation: A "reducing" technique is often adopted for such patients. First strong stimulation on Liming is given until eyeballs are moist or the patients shed tears. If the patients' conditions have improved, the patients will be given needling on the above other acupoints.

4. **痴呆** 常用穴位:天灵、尺桡、中平、脑根、灵宝。

4. Dementia　Frequently-Used Acupoints：Tianling，Chirao，Zhongping，Naogen，Lingbao.

操作：此类患者多为虚证，故多用"补"或"平补平泻"法，若患者已见好转，则转用一般针灸穴位进行治疗。

Operation：Such patients mostly have deficiency syndromes，so "reinforcing" or "even reinforcing and reducing" technique is often used. If the patients'conditions have improved，the patients will be given needling on common acupoints.

5. **失眠**　常用穴位：尺桡、寸桡、中平、胸七，配以百会、三阴交、太冲、申脉、安眠。

5. Insomnia　Frequently-Used Acupoints：Chirao，Cunrao，Zhongping and Xiongqi，in combination with Baihui，Sanyinjiao，Taichong，Shenmai and Anmian.

操作：这种患者多采用"平补平泻"法，给予中等以下强度刺激。

Operation："Even reinforcing and reducing" technique is often adopted for such patients to give stimulation below average.

6. **偏瘫**　常用穴位：中桡、屈委阳、天灵、脑根、灵宝、阴委一、阴委二、阴委三。

6. Hemiplegia　Frequently-Used Acupoints：Zhongrao，Quweiyang，Tianling，Naogen，Lingbao，Yinwei I，Yinwei II and Yinwei III .

操作：此类患者多采用"多泻少补"法，予以强刺激至患者肢体有抽动感为度。

Operation："More-reducing less-reinforcing" technique is often adopted for such patients to give strong stimulation until the patients' limbs have a sense of twitch.

可配以艾炷灸关元和气海，以汗止、脉起、肢温为度。

Moxa-cone moxibustion may be conducted on Guanyuan and Qihai up to stop sweating，arrival of pulsing and warming of limbs.

7. **腰痛**　常用穴位：阴委一、阴委二、阴委三、中平，配以委中透委阳、肾俞透大肠俞、命门透腰俞、太溪透昆仑、肾俞透腰阳关等。

7. Lumbago　Frequently-Used Acupoints：Yinwei I ，Yinwei II ，Yinwei

Ⅲ and Zhongping, in combination with the penetrating through Weizhong to Weiyang, penetrating through Shenshu to Dachangshu, penetrating through Mingmen to Yaoshu, penetrating through Taixi to Kunlun and penetrating through Shenshu to Yaoyangguan.

操作：此类患者多采用补法，寒湿证加灸法，瘀血证局部加拔火罐、委中穴刺络放血。

Operation: A reinforcing technique is often adopted for such patients. For cold-damp syndrome, moxibustion may be added. For syndrome of stasis of blood, fire cupping may be used locally, and bloodletting by pricking Weizhong may be conducted.

四、注意事项

Ⅳ. Precautions

（一）严密消毒
（Ⅰ）Strict Sterilization

透刺时，针锋要经过各种组织层次透达人体深部，所以透刺的消毒，比单刺的消毒要求更为严格。

In acupoint penetration, needle points reach the deep part of the human body through various tissues. Therefore, requirements for sterilization of acupoint penetration are more strict than those for sterilization of single acupuncture.

1. **针具消毒** 用纱布包煮30分钟或高压消毒，临用时需要用75%的酒精棉球拭去针体上沉积的水垢，在急用的情况下，也要用75%的酒精浸泡15分钟。

1. **Sterilization of Needles** The needles are sterilized by boiling gauze-wrapped for 30 minutes or with high pressure sterilization; wipe out water stain on the needle body with 75% alcohol cotton ball before use; for urgent use, immerse the needle with 75% alcohol for 15 minutes.

有条件可用一次性针具。

Use disposable needles if possible.

2. **穴位消毒** 对"透穴"周围皮肤要严格消毒。

2. **Acupoint Sterilization** Strictly sterilize the skin around the "acupoint

penetration".

先用碘酒消毒,然后再用酒精脱碘。

Sterilize with tincture of iodine first, and then use alcohol for deiodination.

刺时勿将针锋穿出"达穴"皮肤之外,出针时易将菌毒带进深部组织而发生感染,如果能够运针自如,只在"透穴"皮肤进行严格消毒也可。

During acupuncture, don't let the needle point penetrate through the skin of "ending acupoint". In needle withdrawal, it is easy to bring bacteria-toxin into the deep tissue and cause infection. If the doctor can handle an operation freely, it is feasible to strictly sterilize the skin around "stroking acupoint".

3. 术者两手消毒　基于刺法需要,不仅持针的右手要接触针体,有时左手也要接触针体辅助进针,故术者两手都要在清洗后,再用碘酒与 75% 的酒精严格消毒。

3. Sterilization of Both Hands of Operators　Based on the need of the acupuncture technique, the right hand of a needle holder contacts the needle body, and sometimes the left hand as an assistant also contacts the needle body to aid in needling. Thus, both hands of the operators should be cleaned and then strictly sterilized with tincture of iodine and 75% alcohol.

(二) 防止折针

(Ⅱ) Prevention for Breaking of Needle

选用较好质量的针,要特别注意固定体位,不要进针过猛。

Select needles with better quality. Pay special attention to the fixed position, and don't insert too quickly.

另外,应注意检查针体,如有残损,不可再用。

In addition, pay attention to inspect the needle body. Don't use a damaged one.

其次,针尖不可过于锋利。

Secondly, the needle point should not be too sharp.

(三) 避免乱针、猛刺与捣针

(Ⅲ) Avoiding actions of Disordering, Jabbing and Thrusting Needles

针刺深度和方向,应随其腧穴分布部位不同而异。

The depths and directions of needling should be changed with different distribution positions of acupoints.

过浅不得气,达不到治疗作用。

If the needles are inserted too shallowly without the arrival of qi, the therapeutic effect cannot be gained.

过深或方向不正确,伤及重要脏器或血管,则会发生意外。

If the needles are inserted too deep or incorrectly in direction, and thus important visceral organs or blood vessels may be injured, thereby causing accidents.

在血管附近的穴位,如果在进针时,手下感觉有波动,则应将针缓慢退出,另换方位刺入。

For acupoints near the blood vessels, if fluctuation is felt under the hand in needling, the needle should be slowly withdrawn and inserted in other positions.

(四) 要随时观察针时的反应
(Ⅳ) Observe Reactions in Acupuncture at All Time

最常见的是休克现象,所以捻针要特别缓慢,且捻且停,随时观察患者的颜面、脉搏、呼吸、血压等变化。

The most common is shock. Therefore, the doctor should twirl the needle body very slowly, twirling the needle while having a brief pause so as to observe change of patient's face, pulse, breath, blood pressure, etc.

若已进入休克前期(意识没有改变)则应起针,令患者卧床休息5~15分钟,即可恢复正常。

If the patient enters the pre-shock stage(no change of consciousness), the doctor should withdraw the needle and let the patient to have a rest in bed for 5-15 minutes until the patient recovers.

但这种现象是治疗所要求的现象,要避免造成严重休克。

But this phenomenon is required for treatment. The operator should avoid causing serious shock.

若出现严重休克,即应首先针刺"寸平"穴(上肢伸侧,腕上一寸,桡侧旁开四分,针五分深有强心提脉之功),其次可针"人中""十宣""合谷"等穴,即可恢复。

94

If the serious shock occurs, first puncture "Cunping" point (on extensor aspect of the upper limbs, 1 cun above the wrist, 4 fen laterally to the radialis; acupuncture for a depth of 5 fen has a function to tonify the heart and to normalize pulse); and then puncture acupoints such as "Renzhong", "Shixuan" and "Hegu", thus the patient will recover.

针后并无任何不良反应。

There is no any adverse reaction after needling.

(五) 施术时的态度
(Ⅴ) Operation Attitudes

术者在接触患者时,尤其是在针刺操作过程中,态度要和蔼、庄重,树立病人对医生的信赖和尊重,使患者乐于接受医生的指导和言语的矫正。

When contacting with the patients, and especially in the operation process of acupuncture, the operator should be affable and solemn and establishes patient's trust and respect on doctors so that the patients are willing to receive guidance and speech correction by the doctors.

(六) 体位选取
(Ⅵ) Position Selection

便于操作,患者舒适,且能较长时间保持稳定的体位,故多取卧位或靠背仰坐位为好,避免隔衣扎针,隔衣扎针不但取穴不准,且无法消毒,更不易掌握深浅。

Select positions which are convenient for operation, comfortable for patients and stable for long time. So it is advisable to select lying positions or sitting position against the backrest. Avoid puncturing through the clothes, which is inaccurate in acupoint selection, impossible for sterilization and difficult in controlling the depth.

五、针刺反应及处理

Ⅴ. Side Reactions and Treatments

休克前期及休克反应:多见于接受重刺激手法体质较弱的患者和对针刺敏感的患者。

Reactions in the pre-shock stage and during shock: This is commonly seen in weak patients receiving strong stimulation and patients sensitive to acupuncture.

主要临床表现为头晕目眩、面色苍白、恶心出汗、血压下降、脉沉细数等。

The major clinical manifestations are dizziness, pale complexion, nausea and perspiration, fall of blood pressure, deep thready and rapid, etc.

处理应立即出针,让患者平卧于床上,经休息或施以针灸治疗后,一般可恢复。

The treatment is to withdraw the needle immediately, and let the patient to supinely lie on the bed. The patient will recover after a rest or acupuncture treatment.

如出现严重的休克或剧烈的呕吐,要随时观察其呼吸、脉搏、血压及意识的变化,必要时需采用吸氧、强心剂、呼吸兴奋剂等救治措施,以防发生意外。

If the patients have a serious shock or severe vomiting, the changes of the patients' breath, pulsation, blood pressure and consciousness must be observed at any time. The emergency measures such as oxygen inhalation, cardiac stimulant and respiratory stimulant should be applied when necessary so as to avoid accidents.

六、针刺后遗反应

Ⅵ. Residual Effect of Acupuncture

1. **中等度刺激可能出现的后遗反应**　全身酸痛、胀麻、下肢发软,单侧或双下肢不全瘫痪,步态跛行。

1. The following residual effects may occur under moderate stimulation Systemic aching, distension and numbness, limpness of lower limbs, incomplete paralysis of one-sided or both lower limbs, and claudication.

一般采用对症处理和针灸治疗,可逐渐恢复。

In general, specific treatment and acupuncture are performed accordingly so as to achieve gradual recovery.

2. **重刺激可能出现的后遗反应**　全身无力,食欲不振,头晕头痛,发热 38~39℃,双下肢软瘫、感觉迟钝,尿潴留或尿失禁等症状。

2. The following residual effects may occur under severe stimulation

General weakness,inappetence,dizziness and headache,fever of about 38-39 ℃,
flaccid paralysis of both lower limbs,dysesthesia,urinary retention or urinary
incontinence.

处理:在卧床恢复阶段要加强护理,防止压疮和肌萎缩。

Handling:Strengthen nursing at the convalescent bedridden stage and prevent
pressure ulcer and amyotrophy.

一般尿潴留,多在 1~3 天内恢复,必要时可导尿。

For general urinary retention,the patient will recover within 1-3 days,and
may be given catheterization when necessary.

七、禁忌证

Ⅶ. Contraindications

1. 极度衰弱营养不良者。

1. Patients who are extremely weak and malnourished.

2. 体温在 38℃以上者。

2. Patients with a body temperature above 38℃.

3. 有严重的并发症者,如非代偿性心脏病、活动性肺结核、糖尿病、急性肾
脏病等。

3. Patients with serious complications,such as non-compensatory heart
disease,active tuberculosis,diabetes,acute kidney disease,etc.

参 考 文 献

References

[1]于涛,包崑.透穴针法临床应用举隅[C]//广东省针灸学会第十二次学术研讨会暨全
国脑卒中及脊柱相关性疾病非药物诊疗技术培训班论文集.广州:广东省针灸学会,
2011:2.

[2]段海涛.过梁针法临床应用[J].四川中医,2002,20(6):72-73.

[3]孙振华.过梁针刺治疗癫狂症 108 例临床分析[J].中国针灸,1995(S2):89-90.

[4]管遵惠.管氏过梁针述要[J].云南中医学院学报,1999(1):3-5.

第二章 灸 法

Chapter 2 Moxibustion

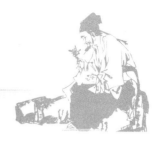

第一节 麦 粒 灸

Section 1 Moxibustion with Seed-Sized Moxa Cone

麦粒灸是使用麦粒大小的艾炷直接放在穴位上烧灼,用以防治疾病的一种疗法,属于直接灸范畴。

Moxibustion with seed-sized moxa cone is a therapy for disease prevention and cure, which is realized through burning the acupoint by putting a seed-sized moxa cone directly on it. It belongs to the category of direct moxibustion.

麦粒灸借助艾火之力,触发机体自我调整功能,是一种具有奇异疗效和特殊生理机制的疗法。

As a therapy with magical curative effects and specific physiological mechanisms, moxibustion with seed-sized moxa cone activates the self-regulation function of the body through the power of the fire from the moxa cone.

具有烟雾小,刺激强,穿透性明显,应用范围广等特点。

It has characteristics of light smoke, strong stimulation, significant penetrability and wide application.

麦粒灸起源于艾炷直接烧灼皮肤的灸法,由中华民族先贤在艾与火结合使用中改良而来,其利用自然资源及生物进化形成的自身调节机制防治疾病。

Moxibustion with seed-sized moxa cone originates from a moxibustion therapy of directly burning the skin with moxa cones. It is an improved therapy made by Chinese sages from combination of moxa cone with fire, which prevents and cures diseases through self-regulation mechanisms formed by natural resources and biological evolution.

但是在历史沿袭中,也许由于有些人不耐直接灸之痛,也许由于操作时耗费人工较多,也许由于缺乏对灸法系统的总结,导致现代人对直接灸了解甚少。

However, in the course of historical inheritance, modern people know little about direct moxibustion, either for some patients cannot stand the pain from the direct moxibustion, or for the operation is time consuming, or for there is not sufficient systematic summarization of moxibustion.

辽宁中医药大学附属医院传统疗法中心对麦粒灸进行深入挖掘整理、改良,现疗效确切,深受患者喜爱(见图 2-1、图 2-2)。

Traditional Therapy Center of Affiliated Hospital of Liaoning University of Traditional Chinese Medicine has carried out deep excavation, systematization and improvement of the moxibustion with seed-sized moxa cone, so the moxibustion therapy has exact curative effects and is favored by patients (See Fig.2-1 and Fig. 2-2).

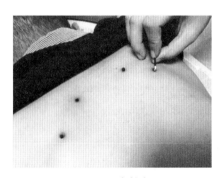

图 2-1 麦粒灸
Fig. 2-1 Moxibustion with seed-sized moxa cone

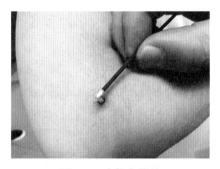

图 2-2 麦粒灸烧灼
Fig. 2-2 Moxa cone burning

一、麦粒灸操作技术

I. Operation of Moxibustion with Seed-Sized Moxa Cone

麦粒灸操作时需要艾绒、油膏、线香、镊子等。

The operation of moxibustion with seed-sized moxa cone needs moxa wool, ointment, joss-sticks, tweezers and so on.

麦粒灸的艾绒要选用存放数年后的艾叶制作,以三年陈艾为佳,其优点是含挥发油少、燃烧缓慢、火力温和,燃着后烟少,艾灰不易脱落,穿透力强,直透皮肤。正如古人形容的"力可穿酒瓮",从而达到理气血、逐寒湿、通经络的效果。

The moxa wool should be made from argy wormwood leaves stored for years, preferably three-year old ones. They have advantages of little volatile oil, slow combustion, moderate fire, little smoke after ignition, uneasy-to-fall-off ash and strong penetrability with the skin penetrated directly, as the ancients said "the power can penetrate the wine jar", thereby regulating qi and blood, dispelling cold-damp and dredging meridians and collaterals.

油膏取其黏附性能,使艾炷稳于体表之上而不倾倒。

For ointment, the adhesion property is focused, so that the moxa cone stands firmly on the body surface without dumping.

麦粒灸艾炷顶部呈尖形,只需要用线香轻轻一触,就能点燃,艾炷顶端越尖越容易点燃,无需明火点燃,以防烧灼皮肤。

The moxa cone for moxibustion with seed-sized moxa cone has a sharp top, which can be ignited by simply a light touch with a joss-stick. The sharper the top of the moxa cone is, the easier it is ignited. However, it should not be ignited by open flame, lest the skin be damaged.

小镊子是用于适时移去残余艾火,并将残余艾火放入盛水的容器里使其熄灭。

The tweezers is used to remove the residual fire in time and put it into a vessel with water for extinguishing.

(一) 灸前准备

(I) Preparation before Moxibustion

1. 艾炷大小的选择 麦粒灸用麦粒作为艾炷形态和大小的标准具有两

方面意义,首先强调麦粒形艾炷的大小,由其高度和腰阔两方面组成,炷高约3mm,腹径 2~3mm,重约 3mg。

1. Choice of Size of Moxa Cone　Considering the seed size as the reference of form and size of moxa cone contains two meanings. Firstly, the emphasis is laid on the size of the seed-sized moxa cone, containing height and waist width, with the height of about 3mm, the abdominal diameter of about 2-3mm, and the weight of about 3mg.

另一方面,麦粒灸会出现难以避免的皮肤烧灼处损伤和由此引发的局部无菌性炎症,以及小型艾炷燃尽时所出现的瞬间烧灼痛(见图 2-3、图 2-4)。

On the other hand, the seed-sized moxibustion will inevitably cause damage to the skin due to burning, thus causing local aseptic inflammation, followed by momentary burning pains due to burning out of small-sized moxa cones (See Fig. 2-3 and Fig. 2-4).

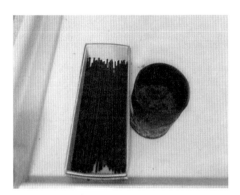

图 2-3　辅助工具

Fig. 2-3　Auxiliary tools

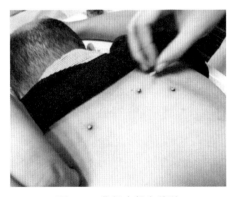

图 2-4　背部麦粒灸烧灼

Fig. 2-4　Burning of moxa cone on the back

2. 选穴、壮数及施灸程度

2. Acupoint Selection, Cone Number and Degree of Moxibustion

（1）施灸选穴

（1）Acupoint Selection

①全身大多数穴位都可施以麦粒灸。

① The seed-sized moxibustion may be applied to most of acupoints throughout the body.

②较多选用背腰、脘腹和下肢等肌肉较厚部位穴位。

② Acupoints on parts with thick muscles such as back, waist, abdomen and lower limbs are mostly selected.

③选穴宜少而精，每次 8~10 穴为宜。

③ Fewer but better acupoints should be selected, preferably 8-10 acupoints each time.

④局部与远部选穴相结合。

④ The acupoints should be selected from both local acupoints and distal acupoints.

⑤定位要准确，以免修正定位造成更多、更大的灸痕。

⑤ The position should be accurate lest more and larger moxibustion marks be caused due to position correction.

⑥分布颜面、血管部位的穴位不可采用化脓瘢痕灸。

⑥ It is unacceptable to apply scarring moxibustion to acupoints on face and ones where there are blood vessels.

（2）施灸壮数：麦粒灸常规灸量每次每穴 1~7 壮。

（2）Cone Number: The conventional quantity of the seed-sized moxibustion should be 1-7 cones per acupoint each time.

具体实施时还需要考虑多方面因素，使壮数与施灸程度协同增效，达到"适宜刺激"的理想程度。

In practice, multiple factors should also be taken into account so that the cone number plays a role together with the degree of moxibustion to reach an ideal degree of "adequate stimulus".

（3）施灸程度：麦粒灸是一种用烧灼来防治疾病的独特方法，灸后穴位局部红晕，属于正常反应，不须处理。

（3）Degree of Moxibustion：Moxibustion with seed-sized moxa cone is a unique method for preventing and curing diseases through burning. After the moxibustion, the acupoint will show blush locally, which is a normal reaction and does not need any treatment.

根据麦粒灸施灸操作强度大小和壮数多寡的不同，在普遍灼痛感觉的基础上，根据局部穴位的不同烧灼程度，还可见黄斑点、小水疱、化脓结痂等多种现象。

On the basis of common burning pain sensation, local acupoints may also show multiple phenomena such as yellow spots, vesicles, suppuration and scabs, depending on the different burning degrees of local acupoints resulting from the operation intensity and cone number of the moxibustion with seed-sized moxa cone.

（二）施灸方法

（Ⅱ）Methods for Moxibustion

1. 非化脓麦粒灸

1. Non-Scarring Moxibustion with Seed-Sized Moxa Cone

（1）解释灸感：向没有麦粒灸经历的患者说明施灸过程和刺激特点，要求患者出现灼痛时立刻呼"烫"，而不要移动肢体，以便及时用镊子捡除残余艾炷，提高患者的依从性，不致因为灼痛乱动肢体，而不能及时移去艾火。

（1）Explaining the moxibustion sensation：Telling unexperienced patients the process and stimulation characteristics of moxibustion, asking them to shout "hot" when the burning pain occurs, instead of moving limbs, so that residual moxa cones can be timely removed with tweezers, thus improving the compliance of patients, lest the fire from the moxa cone cannot be removed due to the limb movement from burning pain.

（2）准备材料：非化脓麦粒灸多采用半粒米样小艾炷，或大半个麦粒样的艾炷,用艾绒制作成软丸或中等硬丸样艾炷。

（2）Preparing materials：The non-scarring moxibustion with seed-sized moxa cone mostly adopts half-grain or more-than-half-grain sized moxa cones，which are soft pill or medium hard pill made from moxa wool.

准备好线香、灭火用盛水小杯、镊子、消毒干棉球、消毒湿棉球等。

Preparing joss-sticks，small cups with water for fire extinguishing，tweezers，sterilized dry cotton balls and sterilized wet cotton balls.

（3）选取体位：使患者处于取穴方便、放松的体位，使体位舒适持久。

（3）Selecting position：The patient is asked in a relaxed position which is easier for acupoint selection，keeping it comfortable and enduring.

注意某些穴位的特殊体位，如施灸膏肓穴，嘱患者两手抱肘，肩胛骨充分展开，使麦粒灸热力透入深部。

Paying attention to special positions for some acupoints，for example，if the moxibustion is applied to the Gaohuang acupoint，the patient should be told to hold elbows with both hands with scapula fully stretched so that the heating power of the moxibustion with seed-sized moxa cone can penetrate deeply.

暴露体位注意防止冷风直接吹拂。

It should be noted that exposed positions are protected from being directly blown by cold wind.

（4）点燃艾炷：在选定的穴位上，用消毒棉签涂上有颜色的中药油膏作为黏附剂。

（4）Igniting moxa cone：Applying colored herbal ointment to the selected acupoint with an aseptic cotton buds as adhesive agent.

将艾炷竖立置于穴位上，用线香暗火点燃艾炷顶端，使其燃烧。

Placing the moxa cone on the acupoint vertically and igniting its top with the smouldering fire of the joss-stick to burn it.

线香接触艾炷之前应将线香积灰掸尽，以防灰烬掉落皮肤，点燃艾炷后的线香搁置于盘中待用。

Before the joss-stick contacts the moxa cone，deposited ashes should be flipped off to prevent ashes falling on the skin，and after the moxa cone is ignited， the joss-stick should be placed in a plate for use.

（5）移除残艾：待艾炷烧剩 2/5~1/5、受试者呼"烫"时，即用镊子将残余艾炷拣到盛水的小杯，再进行下一壮操作。

（5）Removing residual moxa cone：When about 2/5-1/5 of the moxa cone is left and the subject shouts "hot", picking the residual moxa cone with tweezers into a small cup with water, and then starting next cone operation.

软丸样艾炷可以让艾炷在皮肤上自行烧完，当患者感觉灼痛时，用左手拇、食、中指在艾炷四周皮肤略加按压以减轻痛感，软丸样艾炷艾绒量少，因此局部灼痛的时间十分短暂。

A soft pill-like moxa cone may be burnt out on the skin itself. If the patient has a burning pain, slightly pressing the skin around the moxa cone with left thumb, index and middle fingers to alleviate the pain. The soft pill-like moxa cone, because of a small quantity of moxa wool, causes a fairly short local burning pain.

（6）清理皮肤：灸完预定的壮数后，用消毒棉球将穴位处残留灰烬和油膏轻轻擦拭干净，不用涂抹消毒药物。

（6）Cleaning the skin：After the predetermined cone number is completed, slightly wiping off residual ashes and ointment from the acupoints with sterilized cotton balls, without applying sterilizing drugs.

2. 化脓麦粒灸 化脓麦粒灸的操作程序大体与非化脓麦粒灸相似。

2. Scarring Moxibustion with Seed-Sized Moxa Cone The operation of the scarring moxibustion with seed-sized moxa cone is generally similar to that of non-scarring moxibustion with seed-sized moxa cone.

不同之处在于化脓麦粒灸的艾炷多采用艾绒制作成中等硬丸或硬丸样大艾炷或中等麦粒艾炷，对疼痛敏感者艾炷也可由小而逐渐增大，由松而逐渐紧实。

The difference lies in that the moxa cones for scarring moxibustion with seed-sized moxa cone are mostly made from moxa wool into medium hard pills or large hard pill-like moxa cones or medium seed-sized moxa cones, and for pain sensitive group, the moxa cone may be enlarged and tightened gradually.

由于每壮艾炷都要求燃烧完毕,因此刺激程度比非化脓麦粒灸强,施灸后会出现起疱、化脓现象。

Because it is required that each moxa cone be burnt out, the stimulation degree of it is higher than that of non-scarring moxibustion with seed-sized moxa cone, thus showing vesicles and suppuration after the moxibustion.

（1）知情同意:向患者说明化脓灸的作用、操作过程及反应,在患者知情同意前提下实施。

（1）Informed consent:Informing the patient of the function, operation process and reactions of scarring moxibustion, and making implementation on the premise that the patient knows and agrees.

（2）体位舒适:为预防晕灸发生,宜采取卧位或有依靠的坐位。

（2）Comfortable position:In order to prevent fainting during moxibustion, it is preferred that a decubitus position or a well-backed sitting position is taken.

（3）燃尽艾炷:将艾炷竖立置于穴位上,用线香暗火点燃艾炷顶端,使其燃烧。

（3）Burnout of the moxa cone:Placing the moxa cone on the acupoint vertically and igniting its top with the smouldering fire of the joss-stick to burn it.

每壮艾炷燃尽后,掸除艾灰,再安放下一个艾炷继续施灸。

After each moxa cone is burnt out, flipping off the ash to place another moxa cone for next moxibustion.

为减轻患者灼痛,操作者可用手指在灸穴周围皮肤上轻轻按压,并嘱患者张嘴吐气,以转移注意力,松弛肌肉。

In order to alleviate the burning pain of the patient, the operator may press the skin around the acupoint with fingers, and tell the patient to exhale with mouth, in order to divert attention and relax muscles.

（4）清理创面:灸完规定壮数至局部皮肤焦黑,用消毒干棉球将施灸处灰烬轻轻擦拭干净,用消毒干敷料覆盖,不用涂抹消毒药物。

（4）Cleaning the wound surface:After a specified number of cones are completed in such way that local skin is burnt black, slightly wiping off ashes from the acupoints with sterilized dry cotton balls, and covering it with sterilized dry dressings, without applying sterilizing drugs.

（5）灸疮处理：重度麦粒灸之后，往往发生起疱、结痂、溃烂等现象。

（5）Post moxibustion treatment: After a heavy moxibustion, vesicles, scabs and festers often occur.

为了防止摩擦，保护痂皮，预防感染，可用消毒干敷料覆盖。

In order to prevent friction, protect the crusta and prevent the infection, covering it with sterilized dry dressings.

5~7 天后焦痂开始浮动，内有脓样分泌物，可每隔 1~2 天更换敷料，疮口周围用乙醇或盐水棉球揩净，仍用消毒干敷料覆盖，妥善保护灸痂，以便在需要增加脓量继续施灸时，可以在灸痂上施灸，使患者容易忍受灼痛。

5-7 days later, the eschar begins to become unsteady with purulent secretions in it. It is recommended that the dressings be replaced every 1-2 days, and surroundings of the sore be wiped off with cotton balls with alcohol or saline water and covered with sterilized dry dressings again to properly protect the moxibustion scab, so that the moxibustion can be applied to the scab for the patient to endure the burning pain if it is necessary to apply moxibustion again for increasing the amount of the pus.

如发生继发感染，可用黄芩油膏等涂贴，如溃烂面不大，可任其自然结痂恢复。

If a secondary infection occurs, applying and sticking it with scutellaria ointment, and if the fester surface is not large, letting it alone to recover by scabbing naturally.

化脓后 20~30 天，灸疮愈合后形成瘢痕，若瘢痕颜色紫暗或成坚硬疙瘩，还需继续在原处重复施灸。

20-30 days after the fester, the sore will heal up to form a scar, and if the scar presents dark purple or a hard lump, the moxibustion should be applied to the original place again.

若瘢痕颜色灰白，平坦柔软，表明已达到治疗要求。

If the scar presents greyish white, flat and soft, it means that the therapeutic requirements have been met.

二、临床应用

Ⅱ. Clinical Application

（一）适用范围

（Ⅰ）Scope of Application

麦粒灸疗法具有散寒、透热、清毒、扶正的作用,适用于肌肉、骨骼及结缔组织疾病、消化系统疾病、呼吸系统疾病、循环系统疾病、神经系统疾病、泌尿生殖系统疾病,如风湿性关节炎、类风湿关节炎、颈肩腰腿痛、落枕、肩周炎、腹泻、便秘、哮喘、原发性高血压、偏头痛、痛经、月经不调、尿潴留、胃下垂、子宫脱垂、遗尿症、恶性肿瘤等。

The therapy of moxibustion with seed-sized moxa cone has functions of dispelling cold, clearing heat, removing toxicity and strengthening the body resistance, which is applicable to diseases regarding muscles, skeleton and connective tissues, digestive system, respiratory system, circulatory system, nervous system and genitourinary system, such as rheumatic arthritis, rheumatoid arthritis, pains from neck, shoulder, waist and legs, stiff neck, scapulohumeral periarthritis, diarrhoea, constipation, asthma, essential hypertension, hemicrania, dysmenorrhea, menstrual disorders, urinary retention, gastroptosis, hysteroptosis, enuresis and malignant neoplasm.

（二）处方示例

（Ⅱ）Prescription Examples

1. 蛇串疮（带状疱疹） 本病是因肝脾内蕴湿热,兼感邪毒所致。

1. Snake-Like Sores（Herpes Zoster） This disease is caused by dampness-heat in liver and spleen together with toxin infection.

以成簇水疱沿身体一侧带状分布,排列宛如蛇形,且疼痛剧烈为特征的皮肤病。

It is a skin disease which is characterized by zonally-distributed clustering blisters along one side of the body, with a snake-like arrangement and sharp pain.

治法:清热除湿,活血解毒,通络止痛。

Therapeutic Method: Clearing heat and removing dampness, promoting blood circulation to remove toxin and dredging collaterals to stop pain.

选穴：

Acupoint Selection：

主穴：阿是穴（蛇眼、蛇尾）、支沟、阳陵泉。

Major Acupoints：Ashi（snake eye and snake tail）points，Zhigou and Yanglingquan.

配穴：肝经郁火配期门、行间、足窍阴。

Supplement Acupoints：For fire stagnating in liver meridian，adding Qimen，Xingjian and Zuqiaoyin.

脾经湿热配阴陵泉、三阴交、内庭。

For dampness-heat in spleen meridian，adding Yinlingquan，Sanyinjiao and Neiting.

身热加大椎、至阳、合谷。

For body fever，adding Dazhui，Zhiyang and Hegu.

病变在面部三叉神经分布区加风池、听会、太阳、攒竹、外关、合谷。

For lesions on area covered by facial trigeminal nerves，adding Fengchi，Tinghui，Taiyang，Cuanzhu，Waiguan and Hegu.

操作：以最初发疱疹的部位确定两处阿是穴，俗称"蛇眼"穴。

Operation：Determining two Ashi points pointing in the initial position showing herpes，commonly called "snake eye" point.

在疱疹延伸尾端，确定两处阿是穴，俗称"蛇尾"穴。

Determining two Ashi points at the end of the zone along which herpes extend，commonly called "snake tail" point.

治疗过程中，如果"蛇尾"部位继续出现新的红色小疹，可在这些疹点上增加选穴施灸。

During the treatment，if the "snake tail" position still shows new red herpes，additional acupoints may be selected on these herpes for moxibustion.

制作中等硬丸样艾炷。

Preparing medium hard pill-like moxa cones.

患者感觉灼痛可嘱其数数字,或用指压法减痛,当患者感到灼痛十分明显时,即用镊子将残余艾炷夹去。

If the patient feels a burning pain, telling the patient to count or alleviate the pain by finger-pressure method, and if the patient feels a rather obvious burning pain, removing residual moxa cones with tweezers.

按照先"眼"后"尾"的顺序施灸。

The moxibustion should be applied in an order of the "snake eye" before the "snake tail".

每次选用 3~4 穴,每穴施灸 3~9 壮。

3-4 acupoints are selected each time, with 3-9 cones per acupoint.

如四肢远端穴、头面部穴可灸 3 壮,躯体及四肢肌肉丰厚部位穴位可灸 7 壮,疼痛严重部位施灸 7~9 壮,疼痛较轻部位施灸 3~5 壮。

For example, 3 cones for distal acupoints on four limbs and acupoints on head and face, 7 cones for acupoints on positions with thick muscles of body and four limbs, 7-9 cones for severely painful positions and 3-5 cones for slightly painful positions.

急性期每日治疗 1 次,连续治疗 1 周。

In the acute stage, once per day for one week.

后遗症期每周施灸 2~3 次,连续治疗 1~2 个月。

In the sequelae stage, 2-3 times per week for 1-2 months.

2. 肺结核 本病由正气虚弱,感染痨虫,侵蚀肺脏所致。

2. Pulmonary Tuberculosis This disease is caused by deficiency of healthy qi, which results in a tuberculomyces infection in eroded the lung.

表现为咳嗽、咯血、潮热、盗汗及身体逐渐消瘦。

It shows cough, hemoptysis, hectic fever, night sweat and gradual emaciation and weakness.

治法:补虚培元,抗结核杀虫。

Therapeutic Method: Restoring the deficiency and reinforcing the healthy qi to resist and kill the tuberculomyces.

选穴：

Acupoint Selection：

主穴：肺俞、膏肓。

Major Acupoints：Feishu and Gaohuang.

配穴：脾胃虚弱加中脘、足三里。

Supplement Acupoints：For weakness of spleen and stomach，adding Zhongwan and Zusanli.

潮热加大椎、曲池。

For hectic fever，adding Dazhui and Quchi.

咯血加孔最、鱼际。

For hemoptysis，adding Kongzui and Yuji.

操作：制作半粒米软丸样艾炷。

Operation：Preparing half-grain sized soft pill-like moxa cones.

每次选用 2~3 穴，久病、妇幼年老患者灸火不宜太强，感觉灼痛即可移走残艾，每穴施灸 5~7 壮。

2-3 acupoints are selected each time. For chronic patients and women，children and older patients，the fire should not be too strong，and once the patient feels a burning pain，residual moxa cones can be removed，5-7 cones for each acupoint.

新病、壮年患者可采用中等硬丸样艾炷，使艾火灼痛延长少许，再移走残艾，每穴施灸 7~9 壮。

For new patients and postadolescent patients，medium hard pill-like moxa cones may be adopted，and the burning pain caused by the fire should be slightly extended before residual moxa cones are removed. 7-9 cones for each acupoint.

隔日治疗 1 次，治疗 3 个月为 1 个疗程，休息 1 周后，再进入下一疗程施灸，连续施灸 3 个疗程。

One treatment every other day，3 months making a course of treatment，resting for 1 week and then entering next course of moxibustion，keeping for 3 consecutive courses.

3. 哮病(支气管哮喘、喘息性支气管炎) 本病因宿痰内伏于肺,常由外感、饮食、情志、劳倦等诱因而引触,致气滞痰阻,气道挛急、狭窄而发病。

3. Asthma (Bronchial Asthma and Asthmatoid Bronchitis) This disease is caused by latent phlegm retaining in the lung, often induced by external infection, diet, emotion and overstrain, resulting in disease by qi stagnation and phlegm blockade and respiratory tract spasm and narrowness.

发作时喉中哮鸣有声,呼吸气促困难,甚则喘息不能平卧。

In the attacking stage, there is a wheezing in the throat, with a difficult shortness of breath, in severe cases, the patient cannot lie on the back to take breathe.

治法:利气定喘。

Therapeutic Method: Promoting circulation of qi to stop asthma.

发作期攻邪祛痰利气以治标,缓解期补肺、健脾、益肾以治本。

In the attacking stage, treating the symptoms by attacking pathogenic factors to eliminate the phlegm and promote the circulation of qi. In the remission stage, treating the root by tonifying the lung, invigorating the spleen and reinforcing the kidney.

选穴:

Acupoint Selection:

主穴:

Major Acupoints:

发作期:肺俞、膻中、大椎、天突、定喘。

Attacking stage: Feishu, Danzhong, Dazhui, Tiantu and Dingchuan.

缓解期:肺俞、膻中、膏肓、脾俞、肾俞。

Remission Stage: Feishu, Danzhong, Gaohuang, Pishu and Shenshu.

伏灸穴:①肺俞、大椎、风门、定喘。

Acupoints for dog-day moxibustion: ① Feishu, Dazhui, Fengmen and Dingchuan.

②脾俞、心俞、膻中、足三里。

② Pishu, Xinshu, Danzhong and Zusanli.

③肾俞、膏肓、气海、关元。

③ Shenshu, Gaohuang, Qihai, Guanyuan.

配穴：寒饮伏肺配风门、孔最；痰热遏肺配合谷、曲池。

Supplement Acupoints: For cold phlegm-fluid lying latent in the lung, adding Fengmen and Kongzui; and for phlegm-heat inhibiting lung, adding Hegu and Quchi.

操作：每次选用 3~4 穴，先灸背部腧穴，再灸腹部及四肢部腧穴。

Operation: 3-4 acupoints are selected each time, with the moxibustion applied to acupoints on back first and then to acupoints on abdomen and four limbs.

发作期用中等硬丸样艾炷，每次每穴灸 7~9 壮，每日施灸 1~2 次，10 次为 1 疗程。

In the attacking stage, medium hard pill-like moxa cones may be used, with 7-9 cones per acupoint each time, and once to twice per day, 10 times making one course of treatment.

缓解期用半粒米软丸样艾粒，每穴灸 5~7 壮，隔日或隔 2 日 1 次，15~20 次为 1 疗程。

In the remission stage, half-grain sized soft pill-like moxa cones may be used, with 5-7 cones per acupoint, and once every two or three days, 15-20 times making one course of treatment.

第 1 个月隔日 1 次，第 2、3 个月隔 2 天 1 次，可将穴位分为 2~3 组，交替使用，坚持灸 3~6 个月。

In the first month, the moxibustion should be performed once every other day, and in the second and third months, once every three days. The acupoints may be divided into 2-3 groups, which will be used alternatively, persisting for 3-6 months.

4. 慢性泄泻（慢性肠炎、胃肠功能紊乱）　慢性腹泻是由脾虚内生湿滞，肾虚脾失温煦，清浊不分，水谷不化所致。

4. Chronic Diarrhea(Chronic Enteritis and Gastrointestinal Function Disorder)　The chronic diarrhea is caused with result of internal damp-retention, or by deficiency of the spleen and deficiency of the kidney failing to warm the spleen, which makes it unable to separate the clear from the turbid , resulting in undigested foods.

表现排便次数增多,便质稀薄,病程迁延超过 2 个月。

It shows frequent defecation and loose stool, with the course of disease exceeding 2 months.

治法:补肾运脾化湿。

Therapeutic Method: Strengthening the kidney and reinforcing the spleen to remove the dampness.

选穴:

Acupoint Selection:

主穴:气海、天枢、大肠俞、上巨虚。

Major Acupoints: Qihai, Tianshu, Dachangshu and Shangjuxu.

配穴:脾虚加脾俞、足三里。

Supplement Acupoints: For deficiency of the spleen, adding Pishu and Zusanli.

肾虚加关元、命门。

For deficiency of the kidney, adding Guanyuan and Mingmen.

操作:制作半粒米软丸样艾炷。

Operation: Preparing half-grain sized soft pill-like moxa cones.

每次施灸 2~3 穴,每穴 7~9 壮,隔日施灸 1 次,治疗 1 个月为 1 疗程,疗程间隔休息 1 周。连续治疗 3 个月。

The moxibustion should be applied to 2-3 acupoints each time, with 7-9 cones per acupoint and once every other day, 1 month making one course of treatment, at an interval of 1 week between courses for 3 consecutive months.

5. 尪痹(类风湿关节炎) 本病由素体营卫气血不足,外邪乘虚入侵经脉而致。

5. Wangbi(Rheumatoid Arthritis)   This disease is caused by insufficiency of qi, blood, nutritive qi and defensive qi of the body, which makes exogenous pathogenic factor take advantage of a weak point to invade the meridian.

表现为慢性、对称性、多滑膜关节炎和关节外病变,好发于手、腕、足等小关节,常反复发作。

It shows chronic and symmetrical polysynovitis arthritis and extra-articular lesions, which mostly occurs repeatedly in small joints such as hands, wrist and feet.

早期有小关节疼痛、肿胀、晨僵,晚期关节可出现不同程度的僵硬畸形。

In the early stage, there occur pains in small joints, with swellings or morning stiffness, and in the late stage, there may occur different degrees of stiffness or deformations of the joints.

治法:温经止痛。
Therapeutic Method: Warming the meridians to stop pain.

选穴:
Acupoint Selection:

主穴:肾俞、足三里、阿是穴。
Major Acupoints: Shenshu, Zusanli and Ashi points.

配穴:风寒湿阻配大椎、风门。
Supplement Acupoints: For wind-cold-damp retention, adding Dazhui and Fengmen.

风热湿痹配曲池、身柱。
For wind-heat-damp arthralgia, adding Quchi and Shenzhu.

肾阳亏虚配关元、命门。
For deficiency of kidney-yang, adding Guanyuan and Mingmen.

操作:阿是穴常选用疼痛或肿胀最明显点,注意避开血管。
Operation: For Ashi points, points showing the most obvious pains or swellings are often selected, which should avoid blood vessels.

制作半粒米软丸样艾炷,每次施灸 3 个穴位,每穴 7~9 壮,每周施灸 2~3 次,1 个月为 1 疗程,休息 1 周后进入第 2 疗程治疗,共治疗 4~6 个疗程。

Preparing half-grain sized soft pill-like moxa cones, and applying moxibustion to 3 acupoints each time, with 7-9 cones per acupoint and 2-3 times per week, 1 month making one course of treatment, and entering the second course after an interval of 1 week's rest for 4-6 courses.

三、禁忌证

Ⅲ. Contraindication

1. 颜面部、心前区、体表大血管部和关节肌腱部不可用化脓麦粒灸。

1. For facial areas, precordia, larger blood vessels covered by the body surface and muscle tendons of joints, scarring moxibustion with seed-sized moxa cone are not allowed.

2. 妇女妊娠期间,腰骶部和小腹部禁用化脓灸。

2. For pregnant women, scarring moxibustion to lumbosacral areas and hypogastriums are not allowed.

四、注意事项

Ⅳ. Precautions

1. 施行麦粒灸前要给患者解释本技术的操作特点,说明施灸程度和反应,在患者理解和同意后,施行麦粒灸。

1. Before the moxibustion with seed-sized moxa cone, explain the operation characteristics of the technique to the patient, telling the degree and reactions of moxibustion, and implementing the moxibustion with seed-sized moxa cone after the patient knows and agrees.

2. 灸后起疱较小可待其自行吸收,水疱较大者可用消毒针穿破,放出液体,外敷消毒干敷料。

2. After the moxibustion, small vesicles may be left to be absorbed by themselves and big vesicles may be pierced with sterilized needles to release the liquid and covered with sterilized dry dressings.

3. 皮肤感觉迟钝患者,谨慎控制麦粒灸烧灼强度,避免过度灼伤。

3. For patients with insensitive skins, carefully control the burning intensity

of the moxibustion with seed-sized moxa cone, in order to prevent excessive burning.

4. 施行非化脓麦粒灸后可以正常洗浴。

4. After the non-scarring moxibustion with seed-sized moxa cone, the patient may take a bath normally.

化脓麦粒灸的灸疮上，用创可贴盖上后可以洗浴。

Patients with sores resulting from the scarring moxibustion with seed-sized moxa cone may take a bath after the sores are covered with flexible fabric bandages.

洗浴应避免触碰疮面，不要洗脱灸痂。

When taking the bath, do not contact the sore surface, lest the scab be washed off.

长期施行麦粒灸，有疮面、渗出物或结痂者，可用创可贴保护灸疮，采用冲淋，不要过多浸泡和擦洗。

For patients receiving moxibustion with seed-sized moxa cone over a long-term and having sore surfaces, exudations or scabs, flexible fabric bandages may be used to protect sores and a shower may be taken without excessive immersion and scrubbing.

五、意外情况处理方法

V. Treatment for Accidents

灸后皮肤出现红晕是正常现象，若艾火热力过强，施灸过重，皮肤易发生水疱，小水疱无需处理，如果水疱较大用消毒针刺破后消毒，防止感染，数日内可痊愈。

After the moxibustion, the skin may show blushes, which is a normal phenomenon. If the heating power of the fire is too strong, or the moxibustion is applied excessively, the skin is likely to show vesicles. Small vesicles do not need any treatment, and big vesicles should be pierced with sterilized needles and sterilized to protect from infection. These vesicles may be recovered within days.

灸疮化脓期间，正常的无菌性化脓，脓液较淡、色白，若发生细菌感染而化脓,脓液呈黄绿色时,可运用抗生素。

During the suppuration of the sore, if it is an aseptic suppuration, the pus may be light colored and white. If the suppuration occurs due to infection by bacteria, and the pus shows yellowish green, then the antibiotics may be adopted.

假如脓液过多,为防止继发感染,污染衣物,每天可用与皮肤温度相近的生理盐水清洗疮口,并用消毒纱布轻轻擦拭伤口,不要擦伤流血。

If there is too much pus, the sore should be cleaned daily with physiological saline whose temperature is approximate to the skin temperature, in order to prevent secondary infection and clothing contamination, and the wound should be wiped slightly with the sterilized gauze in such a way to avoid scrapping and bleeding.

如疮面不大,20 日左右结痂即可。

If the sore surface is not large, a scab may be formed around 20 days later.

如疮口比较大,要注意脓水的清洗,每日不可间断。

If the sore surface is large, the pus should be cleaned everyday continuously.

参 考 文 献

References

[1] 王玲玲 . 艾灸的特点及温通效应[J]. 中国针灸,2011,31(10):865-868.

[2] 王玲玲 . 麦粒灸临床特点及适宜病症[J]. 上海针灸杂志,2013,32(11):889-891.

[3] 王富春 . 灸法医鉴[M]. 北京:科学技术文献出版社,2009:41-42.

[4] 谢锡亮 . 谢锡亮灸法[M]. 北京:人民军医出版社,2007:63.

[5] 王欣君,王玲玲,张建斌 . 麦粒灸的灸量调控[J]. 上海针灸杂志,2013,32(6):426-429.

[6] 蔡玉梅,郑继范,黄文燕 . 麦粒灸的临床应用和实验研究进展[J]. 针灸临床杂志,
2008,18(9):61-62.

第二节 雷 火 灸

Section 2　Thunder-Fire Moxibustion

雷火灸以经络学说为原理,现代医学为依据,采用纯中药配方,在古代雷

火神针实按灸的基础上,改变其用法与配方创新发展而成的一种疗法。

Thunder-fire moxibustion is a therapy formed by taking the theory of meridians and collaterals as a principle, taking modern medicine as a basis, using a formula of pure Chinese materia medica, and changing the usage and formula thereof on the basis of the pressing moxibustion of ancient thunder-fire wonder moxibustion through innovation and development.

雷火灸为植物药炷,用法为明火悬灸法,灸炷粗约 3cm,具有芳香独特、火力猛、药力峻、渗透力强、治疗范围广等特点,该疗法属于非介入性治疗,治疗时温暖舒适,无毒副作用,无疼痛,治疗效果优于一般艾灸,还能免去患者针刺、吃药、手术的痛苦。

Thunder-fire moxibustion uses vegetable sticks and adopts open fire suspension moxibustion method. The moxibustion wick has a diameter of about 3 cm, and has the characteristics of unique fragrance, strong firepower, powerful medicine efficacy, high permeability, and wide treatment range. The therapy as a non-invasive therapy has the advantages of tenderness and comfort, with no toxic and side effect, no pain, and treatment effect superior to general moxibustion. It can release patients from suffering acupuncture, taking of medicine or surgery.

雷火灸是在古代雷火神针的基础上创新发展而成,首见于李时珍《本草纲目》:"雷火神针法,用熟蕲艾末一两,乳香、没药、穿山甲、硫黄、雄黄、草乌头、川乌头、桃树皮末各一钱,麝香五分,为末,拌艾,以厚纸裁成条,铺药艾于内,紧卷如指大、长三四寸,收贮瓶内,埋地中七七日,取出。用时于灯上点着,吹灭,隔纸十层,乘热针于患处,热气直入病处。"

Thunder-fire moxibustion is formed through innovation and development on the basis of the ancient thunder-fire wonder moxibustion, which appeared in the *Compendium of Materia Medica* written by Li Shizhen for the first time: "In thunder-fire wonder moxibustion, cooked Chinese mugwort powder of 1 liang, frankincense, myrrh, pangolin scales, sulphur, realgar, kusnezoff monkshood root, common monkshood mother root, peach bark powder of 1 qian respectively, and musk of 5 fen in powder are mixed with mugwort. And then the mixture is packed by thick paper to be cut into strips, medicated mugwort is paved in the strips, the strips are twisted into 3 or 4 cun in length as finger, the twisted strips are stored in a bottle, the bottle is buried in the ground and then is taken out after 49 days. While in use, a strip is ignited by a lamp, blown out, and acupunctured on the affected part while it is hot by being insulated by 10 layers of paper, so that hot gas directly enters the affected part."

本法是一种艾灸法,之所以称之为针,是因为操作时,实按于穴位之上,类似于针法之故(见图 2-5、图 2-6)。

This therapy is a moxibustion therapy. The reason of calling it as acupuncture is that in operation, it is actually pressed on acupoint as acupuncture does (see Fig. 2-5 and Fig. 2-6).

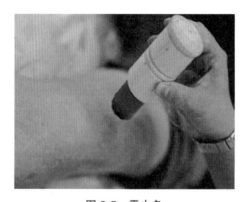

图 2-5 雷火灸
Fig. 2-5 Thunder-fire moxibustion

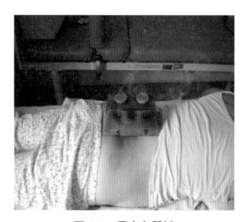

图 2-6 雷火灸器械
Fig. 2-6 Thunder-fire moxibustion instrument

一、雷火灸操作技术

I. Operating Technology of Thunder-Fire Moxibustion

雷火灸是根据人体解剖学的原理,与中医学的脏腑学说、经络学说相结合,通过调节人体组织器官,使之恢复健康状态的一种新的灸疗方法。

Thunder-fire moxibustion is a new moxibustion therapy which is combined with the theory of zang-fu organs and the theory of meridians and collaterals according to the principle of human anatomy and used to adjust human tissues and organs to enable them to restore health.

(一)灸前准备

(I) Preparation Before Moxibustion

1. 选用艾绒 100g,沉香、木香、乳香、茵陈、羌活、干姜、穿山甲各 15g,除艾绒外,其他药物均研为细末,加入麝香少许,调匀。

1. Moxa wool of 100g, and chinese eaglewood, common aucklandia root, frankincense, virgate wormwood herb, incised notopterygium rhizome and root, dried ginger, and pangolin scales of 15g respectively are used, wherein other medicines are all ground into fine powder except moxa wool, a little of musk is added to the powder, and the mixture is fully mixed.

2. 用一尺见方的桑皮纸摊平,将 40g 艾绒和上述药末 10g 调和后均匀铺在纸上。

2. A piece of mulberry paper of one chi square is flattened, moxa wool of 40g and the above-mentioned medicine powder of 10 g are uniformly mixed and then the mixture is paved on the paper.

3. 将桑皮纸卷如爆竹状,外用蛋清涂抹,再糊上桑皮纸一层。

3. The mulberry paper is twisted into firecracker shape, egg white is applied to the outside of the mulberry paper, and then a layer of mulberry paper is pasted on the mulberry paper.

4. 两头留空纸 1 寸许,捻紧即成。

4. Idle paper about 1 cun is respectively left at both ends, and the paper is twisted to form the product.

（二）施灸方法

（Ⅱ）Methods for Moxibustion

1. 雀啄灸法　雷火灸火头对准应灸部位或穴位,火头距离皮肤 1~2cm,形如鸡啄米、雀啄食（见图 2-7）。

1. Bird-Pecking Moxibustion　Fire head of thunder-fire moxibustion aims at the part or acupoint on which moxibustion should be conducted. The head is away from skin at a distance of 1-2cm, and is in the form like chicken pecking rice or bird pecking food（see Fig. 2-7）.

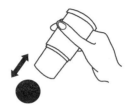

图 2-7　雀啄灸法

Fig. 2-7　Bird-pecking moxibustion

2. 小回旋灸法　雷火灸火头对准应灸的部位或穴位,根据病情需要,火头距离皮肤 1~5cm,做固定的圆弧形旋转,旋转直径 1~3cm（见图 2-8）。

2. Small Revolving Moxibustion　Fire head of thunder-fire moxibustion aims at the part or acupoint on which moxibustion should be conducted. The head is away from skin at a distance of 1-5cm according the patient's condition, and is rotated in fixed circular arc with the rotation diameter of 1-3cm（see Fig. 2-8）.

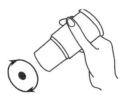

图 2-8　小回旋灸法

Fig. 2-8　Small revolving moxibustion

3. 螺旋灸法　雷火灸火头对准应灸部位中心点,一般火头距离皮肤 2~3cm,做顺时针方向、螺旋式旋转,旋转直径 1~5cm（见图 2-9）。

3. Spiral Moxibustion　Fire head of thunder-fire moxibustion aims at the

center point of the part on which moxibustion should be conducted. The head is away from skin at a distance of 2-3cm, and is clockwise rotated spirally with the rotation diameter of 1-5cm (see Fig. 2-9).

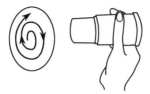

图 2-9 螺旋灸法

Fig. 2-9   Spiral moxibustion

4. 横行灸法 雷火灸火头悬至病灶部位之上,根据病情需要,火头距离皮肤 1~5cm,灸时左右摆动,摆幅为 5~6cm (见图 2-10)。

4. Transverse Moxibustion   Fire head of thunder-fire moxibustion is suspended above the focus part, away from skin at a distance of 1-5cm according the patient's condition, and swung leftwards and rightwards during moxibustion with the swing amplitude of 5-6cm (see Fig. 2-10).

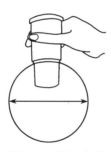

图 2-10   横行灸法

Fig. 2-10   Transverse moxibustion

5. 纵行灸法 雷火灸火头悬至病灶部位之上,根据病情需要,火头距离皮肤 1~5cm,灸时火头沿人体纵轴上下移动,摆幅为 5~6cm (见图 2-11)。

5. Longitudinal Moxibustion   Fire head of thunder-fire moxibustion is suspended above the focus part, away from skin at a distance of 1-5cm according the patient's condition, and moved upwards and downwards along the longitudinal axis of the patient's body during moxibustion with the swing amplitude of 5-6cm (see Fig. 2-11).

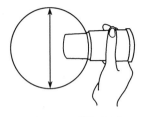

图 2-11 纵行灸法
Fig. 2-11 Longitudinal moxibustion

6. **斜行灸法** 雷火灸火头悬至病灶部位之上,根据病情需要,火头距离皮肤 1~5cm,火头斜行移动,此方法常用于治疗鼻炎等病症,摆幅为 5~6cm(见图 2-12)。

6. **Slant Moxibustion** Fire head of thunder-fire moxibustion is suspended above the focus part, away from skin at a distance of 1-5cm according the patient's condition, and moved slantwise. This method is frequently used to treat rhinitis, and the swing amplitude of 5-6cm(see Fig. 2-12).

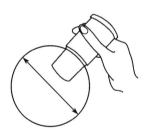

图 2-12 斜行灸法
Fig. 2-12 Slant moxibustion

7. **摆阵法** 用单孔、双孔或多孔斗式温灸盒,根据患者不同病情,在患者身体部位用两个或两个以上的斗式温灸盒平行、斜形或丁字形摆出横阵、竖阵、斜阵、丁字阵等(见图 2-13)。

7. **Array Moxibustion** Bucket type warming moxibustion boxes with single hole, or two holes or multiple holes are used, two or more bucket type warming moxibustion boxes are parallel, slantwise or in T-shape placed on the body part of a patient in a horizontal array, or a vertical array, or a slant array, or a T-shaped array according to the different conditions of patients(see Fig. 2-13).

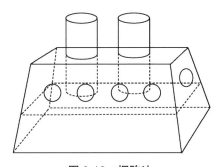

图 2-13 摆阵法
Fig. 2-13 Array moxibustion

二、临床应用

Ⅱ. Clinical Application

(一) 适用范围

(Ⅰ) Scope of Application

雷火灸适用于各类因风寒湿邪侵袭造成的疼痛、麻木等疾病。

Thunder-fire moxibustion is applicable to various pain, numbness and diseases caused by invasion by exogenous pathogenic wind, cold and dampness.

如：

For example：

1. **各类痛疾** 颈椎病、肩周炎、腱鞘炎、网球肘、膝骨性关节炎、腰椎间盘突出症、风湿、骨质增生等。

1. **Various Pain** Such as in cervical spondylosis, scapulohumeral periarthritis, tenosynovitis, tennis elbow, knee osteoarthritis, prolapse of lumbar intervertebral disc, rheumatism, hyperosteogeny, etc.

2. **鼻疾** 急慢性鼻炎、鼻窦炎、变应性鼻炎等。

2. **Nasal Disease** Acute or chronic rhinitis, sinusitis, allergic rhinitis and the like.

3. **眼疾** 眼干燥症、青少年假性近视、弱视、神经性视疲劳、眼上神经痛、眼肌麻痹、结膜炎等。

3. **Eye Disease** Xerophthalmia, adolescent pseudomyopia, amblyopia, nervous asthenopia, ocular neuralgia, ophthalmoplegia, conjunctivitis and the like.

4. 耳喉疾病　耳鸣、突发性耳聋、慢性咽炎等。

4. Ear and Throat Diseases　Tinnitus, sudden deafness, chronic pharyngitis and the like.

5. 妇科疾病　痛经、输卵管炎、卵巢囊肿、子宫肌瘤、乳腺增生等。

5. Gynecological Diseases　Dysmenorrhea, salpingitis, ovarian cyst, hysteromyoma, hyperplasia of mammary glands and the like.

6. 男性疾病　前列腺炎初期、尿失禁、阳痿等。

6. Male Diseases　Primary prostatitis, urinary incontinence, impotence and the like.

7. 消化系统疾病　肠炎、胃炎、各种腹泻和虚寒型便秘等。

7. Digestive System Diseases　Enteritis, gastritis, various diarrhoea and deficiency-cold type constipation and the like.

8. 肥胖症　单纯性肥胖、局部肥胖、产后肥胖等。

8. Obesity　Simple obesity, local obesity, postpartum obesity and the like.

9. 亚健康调理　失眠、手术后康复治疗、亚健康保健等。

9. Sub-Health Conditioning　Insomnia, postoperative rehabilitation, sub-health care and the like.

（二）处方示例

（Ⅱ）Prescription Examples

1. 能近怯远（青少年近视）　多因先天禀赋不足、劳伤心神，或久视伤血，使心肝气血受损，或用眼习惯不良，如看书、写字距离太近，坐位姿势不正及光线过强或不足等，使目络瘀阻，目失所养，导致本病。

1. Shortsightedness (Teenagers' Myopia)　This disease is mainly caused by congenital deficiencies, or internal lesion due to overexertion of mind, or impairment of blood by looking for a long time, which leads to damage to heart and liver, or bad eye care habits such as near distance between eyes and book/paper, incorrect sitting position and excessive/insufficient lighting, which lead to stagnation in the collaterals of eye and eye malnutrition.

表现为看远处模糊，看近处清楚。

The manifestation is blurred vision for objects far away and clear vision for objects nearby.

治法：舒筋活血。

Treatment Method：Relieving rigidity of muscles and promoting blood circulation.

灸法：雀啄、小回旋、横行、螺旋灸法。

Moxibustion Methods：Bird-pecking moxibustion，small revolving moxibustion，transverse moxibustion and spiral moxibustion.

部位：双眼、额头、双耳。

Moxibustion Parts：Eyes，forehead and ears.

穴位：睛明、鱼腰、瞳子髎、四白、合谷。

Acupoints：Jingming，Yuyao，Tongziliao，Sibai and Hegu.

真性近视加灸风池、风府、大椎、肝俞。

Moxibustion is additionally performed on Fengchi，Fengfu，Dazhui and Ganshu for true myopia.

操作：患者取坐位（头直立勿仰，以免火灰掉入眼内）。

Operation：The patient should take a sitting position（keep the head upright but don't look up to prevent fire ash from falling into the eyes）.

按下列顺序操作：

Operate in the following sequence：

（1）用横行灸法灸双眼：双眼闭合，火头距离皮肤 2~3cm，在双眼部来回平行摆动，每来回摆动 10 次为 1 壮，每灸 1 壮用手按压眼部 1 次。

（1）The transverse moxibustion is performed on both eyes：The patient should close both eyes，the fire head is away from skin at a distance of 2-3cm and is swung back and forth in parallel to the eyes，swinging back and forth 10 times is used as 1 zhuang，and the eyes are pressed once by hand when moxibustion is performed for 1 zhuang.

灸至皮肤发红、结膜充血为度。

Moxibustion is preformed till skin becomes red and conjunctiva becomes congestive.

（2）用雀啄法灸睛明、鱼腰、瞳子髎、四白,火头距离皮肤约 2cm,每雀啄 8 次为 1 壮,每灸 1 壮用手按压穴位 1 次,每穴灸 4~6 壮。

（2）The bird-pecking moxibustion is performed on Jingming, Yuyao, Tongziliao and Sibai, the fire head is away from skin at a distance of 2cm, bird-pecking of 8 times is used as 1 zhuang, the acupoints are pressed once by hand when moxibustion is performed for 1 zhuang, and moxibustion is performed on each acupoint for 4-6 zhuangs.

（3）用横行灸法灸双眼、额部:双眼张开,平视前方,火头距离皮肤 2~3cm,在双眼部来回平行移动,每来回移动 10 次为 1 壮,每壮之间嘱患者闭眼,术者用手按压双眼一次,共灸 8 壮。

（3）The transverse moxibustion is performed on both eyes and forehead:The patient should open both eyes and look at the front horizontally, the fire head is away from skin at a distance of 2-3cm and is moved back and forth in parallel to the eyes, moving back and forth 10 times is used as 1 zhuang. The patient should be told to close eyes and the moxibustion performer should press the eyes once by hand between every two zhuangs, and moxibustion is performed for 8 zhuangs in total.

距离额部皮肤 2~3cm 来回平行移动,每来回移动 10 次为 1 壮,灸 10 壮。

The fire head is away from the skin of forehead at a distance of 2-3cm and is moved back and forth in parallel, moving back and forth 10 times is used as 1 zhuang, and moxibustion is performed for 10 zhuangs.

（4）用螺旋灸法灸耳郭正面、背面:火头距离皮肤 2~3cm,每旋转 8 次为 1 壮,每壮之间用手按压一下,灸至耳郭正面、背面发红为度。

（4）The spiral moxibustion is performed on the front and back sides of the auricle:The fire head is away from skin at a distance of 2-3cm, rotation of 8 times is used as 1 zhuang, pressing is preformed once by hand between every two zhuangs, and moxibustion is performed till the front and back sides of the auricle become red.

（5）用雀啄法灸外耳道口:火头距离外耳道口 2cm,雀啄 8 次为 1 壮,左右各灸 3 壮。

（5）The bird-pecking moxibustion is performed on external auditory canal opening:The fire head is away from external auditory canal opening at a distance of 2cm, bird-pecking of 8 times is used as 1 zhuang, and moxibustion is performed on each external auditory canal opening for 3 zhuangs.

（6）重复操作步骤（1）。

（6）Repeat step（1）.

（7）雀啄法灸合谷 4 壮，雀啄 8 次为 1 壮，距离皮肤 2cm。

（7）The bird-pecking moxibustion is performed on Hegu for 4 zhuangs, bird-pecking of 8 times is used as 1 zhuang, and the fire head is away from skin at a distance of 2cm.

（8）真性近视加灸风池、风府、大椎、肝俞，各灸 8 壮，用回旋灸法，回旋 8 次为 1 壮，距离皮肤 2cm。

（8）Moxibustion is additionally performed on Fengchi, Fengfu, Dazhui and Ganshu for true myopia. The revolving moxibustion is performed on each acupoint for 8 zhuangs, revolving of 8 times is used as 1 zhuang, and the fire head is away from skin at a distance of 2cm.

灸疗完毕，患者闭目休息 3 分钟。

Let the patient close his/her eyes and have a rest for 3 minutes after moxibustion.

每日灸治 1 次，每周为一疗程，疗程间休息 1 天，一般灸治 2~5 个疗程。

Moxibustion is performed once every day, and 10 times make a treatment course. There should be a one-day rest between two treatment courses, and moxibustion is usually performed for 2-5 treatment courses.

视力恢复正常后可做每周 1 次的巩固性治疗。

Consolidation treatment can be performed once every week after the sight is restored to normal.

成年近视患者采用本法灸疗，可稳定视力。

This moxibustion may be used for adult myopia patients to stabilize their sight.

提示：治疗期间注意用眼卫生。

Note：Patients should pay attention to eye hygiene during the treatment.

2.**神水将枯(眼干燥症)**　本病多因脾胃阳虚,不能生化水谷精微,或肝肾阴虚,气血不足,或风邪犯肺,目失濡养而发生的眼部疾病,表现为眼干涩胀痛、视力下降等症状。

2. **Dry Eye Syndrome(Xerophthalmia)**　This disease is an eye disease mainly due to that the eyes lose their nutrients,which is caused by yang deficiency of the spleen and stomach being unable to digest and absorb the essence of water and grain,or yin deficiency of the liver and kidney and deficiency of qi and blood, or pathogenic wind invading the lung. The manifestation includes dryness and distending pain of eyes,fading eyesight,etc.

治法:舒筋活络。

Treatment Method:Relieving rigidity of muscles and activating collaterals.

灸法:横行、螺旋、小回旋、雀啄灸法。

Moxibustion Methods:Transverse moxibustion,spiral moxibustion,small revolving moxibustion,and bird-pecking moxibustion.

部位:额部、双眼、双耳。

Moxibustion Parts:Forehead,eyes and ears.

穴位:睛明、翳风、合谷、眼(耳穴)。

Acupoints:Jingming,Yifeng,Hegu and Yan(an auricular acupoint).

操作:患者取坐位(头直立勿仰,以免火灰掉入眼内)。

Operation:The patient should take a sitting position(keep the head upright but don't look up to prevent fire ash from falling into the eyes).

(1)用横行灸法灸前额部:火头距离皮肤 2~3cm,在前额部发际与眉部边缘之间做横行移动,每横行 10 次为 1 壮,每灸 1 壮用手按压额部 1 次,灸至皮肤发红、发热为度。

(1) The transverse moxibustion is performed on forehead:The fire head is away from skin at a distance of 2-3cm and moved transversely between the hair line and eyebrows on the forehead,transverse moving of 10 times is used as 1 zhuang,the forehead is pressed once by hand when moxibustion is performed for 1 zhuang,and moxibustion is performed till skin becomes red and warm.

(2)用横行灸法灸双眼部:双眼闭合,火头距离皮肤 2~3cm,在双眼部来回平行移动,每来回 10 次为 1 壮,每灸 1 壮用手按压眼部 1 次,灸至皮肤发红、结膜充血为度。

(2) The transverse moxibustion is performed on both eyes:The patient should close both eyes,the fire head is away from skin at a distance of 2-3cm and moved back and forth in parallel to the eyes,moving back and forth 10 times is used as 1 zhuang,the eyes are pressed once by hand when moxibustion is performed for 1 zhuang,and moxibustion is performed till skin becomes red and conjunctiva becomes congestive.

(3) 用小回旋法灸双眼:双眼睁开,火头距离眼部 2~3cm,顺时针旋转灸双眼,速度适中,眼球不动,每回旋 10 次为 1 壮,每壮之间嘱患者闭眼,术者用手按压双眼 1 次,灸 10 壮。

(3) The small revolving moxibustion is performed on both eyes:The patient should open both eyes,the fire head is away from eyes at a distance of 2-3cm and revolved clockwise to perform moxibustion on both eyes with a moderate speed and with eyeballs keeping stationary,revolving of 10 times is used as 1 zhuang, the patient should be told to close eyes and the moxibustion performer should press the eyes once by hand between every two zhuangs,and moxibustion is performed for 10 zhuangs.

(4) 用雀啄法灸睛明:火头距离皮肤 2~3cm,每雀啄 10 次为 1 壮,每壮之间用食指揉按 1 次,灸 8 壮。

(4) The bird-pecking moxibustion is performed on Jingming:The fire head is away from skin at a distance of 2-3cm,bird-pecking of 10 times is used as 1 zhuang,the acupoint is pressed once by forefinger between every two zhuangs, and moxibustion is performed for 8 zhuangs.

(5) 用横行灸法灸双眼:双眼睁开,火头距离皮肤 2~3cm,火头横行来回移动,每来回移动 10 次为 1 壮,每壮之间用手按压眼部,灸 8 壮。

(5) The transverse moxibustion is performed on both eyes:The patient should open both eyes,the fire head is away from skin at a distance of 2-3cm and moved back and forth transversely,moving back and forth 10 times is used as 1 zhuang, and the eyes are pressed by hand between every two zhuangs,and moxibustion is performed for 8 zhuangs.

（6）用螺旋灸法灸双耳：火头距离皮肤 2~3cm，灸至双耳发红、发热为度。

（6）The spiral moxibustion is performed on both ears：The fire head is away from skin at a distance of 2-3cm，and moxibustion is performed till the ears become red and warm.

（7）用雀啄法依次点灸外耳道口、眼（耳穴）、翳风，火头距离皮肤约 2cm，每雀啄 10 次为 1 壮，每壮之间用手压 1 次，各灸 8 壮。

（7）The bird-pecking moxibustion is performed successively on external auditory canal opening，Yan（an auricular acupoint）and Yifeng. The fire head is away from skin at a distance of 2cm，bird-pecking of 10 times is used as 1 zhuang，pressing is performed once by hand between every two zhuangs，and moxibustion is performed for 8 zhuangs at each position.

（8）用雀啄法灸合谷：火头距离皮肤 2~3cm，雀啄 10 次为 1 壮，每壮之间用手按压 1 次穴位，灸 8 壮。

（8）The bird-pecking moxibustion is performed on Hegu：The fire head is away from skin at a distance of 2-3cm，bird-pecking of 10 times is used as 1 zhuang，the acupoint is pressed once by hand between every two zhuangs，and moxibustion is performed for 8 zhuangs.

每日灸疗 1 次，10 天为 1 疗程，一般灸 3~5 个疗程，每疗程间休息 1 天。

Moxibustion is performed once every day，and 10 times make a treatment course. Moxibustion is usually performed for 3-5 treatment courses，and there should be a one-day rest between two treatment courses.

提示：治疗期间眼底出血禁灸。

Note：Do not perform moxibustion if the patient has fundus hemorrhage during the treatment.

3. **鼻鼽（变应性鼻炎）** 本病多由肺气虚弱，脾肾虚损，卫表不固，腠理疏松，风寒湿邪乘虚而入，邪气相搏，肺气不宣，侵犯鼻窍所致。

3. Allergic Rhinitis（Anaphylactic Rhinitis） This disease is resulting from obstruction of lung qi invading nasal orifices，which is mainly caused by insufficiency of lung qi，impairment of the spleen and kidney，failure of defensive qi to protect the body，looseness of the striae of the skin and muscles，and thus pathogenic wind，cold and dampness invade the body by taking advantage of weak

body resistance.

临床主要表现为喷嚏、鼻塞、鼻痒、流涕等。

The clinical manifestations include sneezing, nasal obstruction, rhinocnesmus, watery nasal discharge, etc.

治法:疏风祛邪,通窍固表。

Treatment Method: Expelling wind to eliminate pathogenic factors, and dredging nasal orifices and consolidating the defensive qi.

灸法:纵行、斜行、雀啄、螺旋、横行灸法。

Moxibustion Methods: Longitudinal moxibustion, slant moxibustion, bird-pecking moxibustion, spiral moxibustion, and transverse moxibustion.

部位:上星至素髎部、印堂至迎香部、耳部、额部。

Moxibustion Parts: Segment from Shangxing to Suliao, segment from Yintang to Yingxiang, ears, and forehead.

穴位:上星、素髎、睛明、印堂、迎香、列缺、合谷。

Acupoints: Shangxing, Suliao, Jingming, Yintang, Yingxiang, Lieque and Hegu.

操作:患者取坐位(头直立勿仰,以免火灰掉入眼内)。

Operation: The patient should take a sitting position (keep the head upright but don't look up to prevent fire ash from falling into the eyes).

(1) 用纵行法灸上星至素髎部:火头距离皮肤2~3cm,上下灸10次为1壮,每壮灸完后用手按一下,共灸60壮。

(1) The longitudinal moxibustion is performed on the segment from Shangxing to Suliao: The fire head is away from skin at a distance of 2-3cm, moving up and down for 10 times is used as 1 zhuang, pressing is performed once by hand when moxibustion is performed for 1 zhuang, and moxibustion is performed for 60 zhuangs in total.

(2) 用斜行法灸印堂至迎香部:做"八"字斜行灸,操作方法同上。

(2) The slant moxibustion is performed on the segment from Yintang to Yingxiang: The moxibustion is performed by moving the fire head in an inverted-V

pattern, and the operating method is the same as above.

（3）用横行法灸额部：火头距离皮肤 2~3cm，在额部发迹与眉部边缘之间做横行移动，横行 10 次为 1 壮，共灸 3 壮。

（3）The transverse moxibustion is performed on forehead: The fire head is away from skin at a distance of 2-3cm and moved transversely between the hair line and eyebrows on the forehead, transverse moving of 10 times is used as 1 zhuang, and moxibustion is performed for 3 zhuangs in total.

（4）用雀啄法灸印堂、睛明、迎香、上星：火头距离皮肤 2~3cm，雀啄 10 次为 1 壮，每壮之间用手按压一下，每穴各灸 5 壮，12 岁以下的患者每穴灸 3 壮。

（4）The bird-pecking moxibustion is performed on Yintang, Jingming, Yingxiang and Shangxing: The fire head is away from skin at a distance of 2-3cm, bird-pecking of 10 times is used as 1 zhuang, pressing is performed once by hand between every two zhuangs, and moxibustion is performed for 5 zhuangs on each acupoint, or 3 zhuangs on each acupoint for patients under 12 years old.

（5）用螺旋法灸耳郭正面、背面：火头距离皮肤 2~3cm，螺旋 10 次为 1 壮，每壮之间用手压一下，灸至耳郭发红。

（5）The spiral moxibustion is performed on the front and back sides of the auricle: The fire head is away from skin at a distance of 2-3cm, rotation of 10 times is used as 1 zhuang, pressing is preformed once by hand between every two zhuangs, and moxibustion is performed till the auricle becomes red.

（6）用雀啄法灸外耳道口：牵拉耳郭，使外耳道口充分暴露，雀啄 10 次为 1 壮，每壮之间用手压一下，两外耳道口各灸 3~5 壮。

（6）The bird-pecking moxibustion is performed on external auditory canal opening: The auricle is pulled to expose the external auditory canal, bird-pecking of 10 times is used as 1 zhuang, pressing is preformed once by hand between every two zhuangs, and moxibustion is performed on each external auditory canal opening for 3-5 zhuangs.

（7）用雀啄法灸鼻孔：指压上唇，火头距离鼻孔 2cm，同时让病人头后仰做深呼吸，雀啄 10 次为 1 壮，共灸 3 壮，12 岁以下者可灸 2 壮。

（7）The bird-pecking moxibustion is performed on nostrils:The upper lip is pressed by a finger,the fire head is away from nostrils at a distance of 2cm, meanwhile,let the patient tilt his/her head back and take a deep breath,bird-pecking of 10 times is used as 1 zhuang,and moxibustion is performed for 3 zhuangs in total,or 2 zhuangs in total for patients under 12 years old.

（8）用雀啄法灸列缺、合谷:火头距离皮肤 2~3cm,雀啄 7 次为 1 壮,每壮之间用手压一下,每穴灸 3 壮。

（8）The bird-pecking moxibustion is performed on Lieque and Hegu:The fire head is away from skin at a distance of 2-3cm,bird-pecking of 7 times is used as 1 zhuang,pressing is performed once by hand between every two zhuangs,and moxibustion is performed for 3 zhuangs on each acupoint.

整个操作过程约25分钟,每天1次或2次,7天为1疗程,疗程间休息1天,治疗 3 个疗程。

The whole operating procedure takes about 25 minutes. Moxibustion is performed 1 or 2 times every day,and 7 times make a treatment course. There should be a one-day rest between two treatment courses,and moxibustion should be performed for 3 treatment courses.

提示:鼻部出血禁灸。
Note:Do not perform moxibustion if the patient has nosebleed.

4.腰痛病(腰椎间盘突出症) 本病多因身体素虚,肾精亏损,致骨失所养,或劳作过度、运动失当,致腰腿疼痛。

4. Lumbago(Prolapse of Lumbar Intervertebral Disc) The manifestation of this disease is mainly resulting from bone malnutrition caused by weak constitution and kidney essence deficiency,or waist and leg pain caused by overwork and inappropriate movement.

遇寒、暑、湿邪气侵犯腰腿部时,可加重或诱发本病。
This disease may be worsened or induced when waist and legs are invaded by pathogenic cold,heat,and dampness.

治法:温经活络,散寒止痛。
Treatment Method:Warming meridians and activating collaterals,and

eliminating cold to stop pain.

灸法：回旋、横行、摆阵灸法。

Moxibustion Methods：Revolving moxibustion，transverse moxibustion and array moxibustion.

部位：腰椎及腰骶椎部、患侧臀部。

Moxibustion Parts：Lumbar vertebra，lumbosacral vertebrae and buttock of affected side.

穴位：环跳、委中。

Acupoints：Huantiao and Weizhong.

操作：患者俯卧病床。

Operation：The patient should lie prone in the bed.

（1）摆阵法：双孔或多孔斗式灸具，置灸盒于腰椎、腰骶关节，盖上浴巾，温灸 30~40 分钟，每 15 分钟吹药灰 1 次。

（1）Array Moxibustion：The bucket type moxibustion boxes with two holes or multiple holes are used，the moxibustion boxes are placed on the lumbar vertebra and lumbosacral joint and covered with a bath towel，warming moxibustion is performed for 30-40 minutes，and medicine ash is blown once every 15 minutes.

（2）悬灸法：火头距离皮肤 2~3cm，用横行法灸患侧臀部疼痛部位，灸至皮肤发红、发热，灸 10 次用手压一下。

（2）Suspension Moxibustion：The fire head is away from skin at a distance of 2-3cm，the transverse moxibustion is performed on the pain part of the buttock of the affected side till skin becomes red and warm，and pressing is performed once by hand when moxibustion is performed for 10 times.

（3）悬灸点穴法：火头距离皮肤 2~3cm，用回旋法灸环跳、委中，回旋 10 次为 1 壮，每灸 1 壮，用手压一下，每穴位各灸 8 壮。

（3）Suspension Moxibustion and Finger Pointing Manipulation：The fire head is away from skin at a distance of 2-3cm，the revolving moxibustion is performed on Huantiao and Weizhong，revolving of 10 times is used as 1 zhuang，pressing is performed once by hand when moxibustion is performed for 1 zhuang，and moxibustion is performed on each acupoint for 8 zhuangs.

下肢酸胀疼痛麻木部位,用左手平压腰部并向下滑动,火头随指尖移动,距离皮肤 2cm,滑动 10 次为 1 壮,共灸 7~9 壮。

For sore, swollen, pain and numb part of lower limbs, horizontally press the waist by the left hand and then slide it downwards, the fire head is moved along with the fingertip and is away from skin at a distance of 2cm, slide of 10 times is used as 1 zhuang, and moxibustion is performed for 7-9 zhuangs in total.

每天灸 1 次,10 天为 1 疗程,可连续灸 1~2 个疗程,若有腰椎滑脱等其他合并症,可灸 3~5 个疗程。

Moxibustion is performed once every day. 10 times make a treatment course. Moxibustion may be continuously performed for 1-2 treatment courses. If the patient has lumbar spondylolisthesis and other complication, moxibustion may be performed on him/her for 3-5 treatment courses.

三、禁忌证

Ⅲ. Contraindications

眼外伤、青光眼、眼底出血、发热、脑血管病急性期、高血压危象及妊娠等患者禁用。

Do not use for patients with ocular trauma, glaucoma, fundus hemorrhage, fever, cerebrovascular disease in acute phase, hypertensive crisis, and pregnant women.

四、注意事项

Ⅳ. Precautions

1. 用灸时,火头应与皮肤保持适当距离,以患者能耐受为度,切忌火头接触皮肤,以免烫伤。

1. When moxibustion is used, keep appropriate distance between the fire head and skin by taking the distance capable of being endured by the patient as a standard. Do not contact skin by fire head to avoid scalding.

如有皮肤烫灼伤,应对症处理。

If skin has scalds or burns, specific treatment should be performed accordingly.

2. 治疗过程中应注意用火安全,避免火灾发生。

2. Pay attention to fire safety during the treatment to prevent fire.

3. 治疗后,2 小时内勿擦洗灸疗部位,否则影响疗效。

3. Do not wipe and wash the part on which moxibustion treatment is performed within 2 hours after treatment. Otherwise, treatment effect may be affected.

五、意外情况处理方法

V. Treatment for Accidents

如出现心悸、血压升高等情况时应马上停止治疗,嘱患者平躺静卧检测血压,如症状不缓解要对症给药治疗。

If the conditions such as palpitation and rise in blood pressure appear, stop treatment immediately, tell the patient to lie flat and repose, and then the patient's blood pressure should be tested. Specific treatment should be performed accordingly if the symptoms are not relieved.

注意患者状态、感觉,治疗时认真调节温度,防止烫伤发生。

Pay attention to the state and feeling of the patient. Carefully adjust temperature during treatment to prevent scalding.

如果出现烫伤马上停止治疗,并在烫伤处消毒涂抹烫伤药。

Immediately stop treatment if scalds appear, and sterilize and apply medicine for treating scald.

参 考 文 献

References

[1] 薛昊,郭静,赵占豪,等.雷火神针热传递特性的实验研究[J].上海针灸杂志,2016,35(6):745-750.

[2] 蔡树河,丁怀利,吴炳煌,等.关于艾灸治疗中"火候"的认识[J].中国中医药现代远

程教育,2015,13(15):63-64.

[3] 刘树正,王阳,陈鹏.雷火灸临床应用概况[J].实用中医药杂志,2015,31(4):362-365.

[4] 廖秋菊,张芸.赵氏雷火灸临床应用概述[J].实用中医药杂志,2014,30(6):575-577.

[5] 周建伟.《肘后备急方》急症灸治探讨[J].针灸临床杂志,1996,6(12):9-10.

[6] 赵源.灸法的临床应用及机理探讨[J].中国针灸,1995,12(2):47-48.

第三节 隔 物 灸
Section 3 Indirect Moxibustion

隔物灸,指施用灸法时,将艾炷或艾条放置在姜片(隔姜灸)、蒜片(隔蒜灸)、食盐(隔盐灸)或药品制成的薄饼(附子饼灸等)上施灸的方法,又称隔药灸。

Indirect moxibustion, also known as herb-partitioned moxibustion, refers to the method in which the moxa cone or moxa stick is placed on the ginger slices (ginger moxibustion), garlic slices (garlic moxibustion), salt (salt moxibustion) or thin cakes made of medicine (such as monkshood cake moxibustion) for moxibustion.

隔物灸不仅有艾灸温经散寒、活血通脉、消瘀散结及防病保健的作用,还具有所选用药物的治疗作用,在临床上应用广泛。

The indirect moxibustion not only has the effect of warming meridians to dissipate cold, promoting blood circulation to dredge collaterals, dispersing blood stasis to dissolve lumps in addition to disease prevention and health care, but also has the therapeutic effect of the selected drugs. So it is widely used clinically.

隔物灸是我国古代劳动人民在长期与疾病作斗争的过程中创造的一种疗法。

Indirect moxibustion is a kind of therapy created by the ancient Chinese working people in their long-term struggle with the disease.

最早出现于东晋·葛洪所著的《肘后备急方》。

It first appeared in the *Handbook of Prescription for Emergency* by Ge Hong in the Eastern Jin Dynasty.

隔物灸对各系统多种疾病有确切疗效,尤以隔姜灸、复方隔物灸的应用更为多见。

Indirect moxibustion is effective against multiple diseases in different systems. Especially the application of ginger moxibustion and compound indirect moxibustion is more common.

一、隔物灸操作技术

Ⅰ. Operation Techniques of Indirect Moxibustion

隔物灸也叫间接灸、间隔灸,是利用药物等材料将艾炷和穴位皮肤隔开施灸的一种操作技术。

The indirect moxibustion is also called indirect moxibustion or partition moxibustion, which is a kind of operation technique in which moxibustion is given by separating the moxa cone from the skin of the acupoint with medicine.

隔物灸可以避免灼伤皮肤,还能借间隔物的药力和艾炷的特性发挥协同作用,以取得更佳效果。

The indirect moxibustion can prevent the skin from burning and there can also appear a synergetic effect by the potency of the spacer and the characteristics of the moxa cone to achieve better results.

临床上可用于治疗多种疾病,特别是证属虚寒性的疾病。

Clinically, it can be used to treat a variety of diseases, especially those with cold syndrome of deficiency type.

(一) 灸前准备

(Ⅰ) Preparation before Moxibustion

1. 艾炷制备

1. Preparation of Moxa Cone

艾绒制备:取陈艾叶经过反复晒干,筛拣干净,除去杂质,令软细如棉,即称为艾绒。

Preparation of Moxa wool: The stockpiled argy wormwood leaves are sunbaked repeatedly with impurities removed by sifting, which makes it as soft as cotton.

艾炷制备:艾绒做成圆锥形状之小团,称为艾炷,艾炷燃烧一枚,称为一壮。

Preparation of Moxa Cone: A small wad made from moxa wool is called moxa cone, and a burnt moxa cone is called one zhuang.

2. 间隔物制备
2. Preparation of Spacers

根据病情制作不同的间隔物,如姜片、蒜片、食盐及药饼等,并在其上用针点刺小孔若干。

According to the patient's condition, different spacers should be made, such as ginger slices, garlic slices, salt and medicated cake, on which quick puncture is performed with a needle, forming several tiny holes.

(二) 施灸方法
(Ⅱ) Methods for Moxibustion

1. 隔姜灸 选取整块新鲜生姜,纵切成 2~3mm 厚度的姜片,在其上用针点刺小孔若干。

1. Ginger Moxibustion The whole piece of fresh ginger is selected and lengthwise cut into ginger slices of 2-3mm in thickness, on which quick puncture is performed with a needle, forming several tiny holes.

施灸时,将一底面直径约 10mm、高约 15mm 的圆锥形艾炷放置姜片上,从顶端点燃艾炷,待快燃烧尽时在上面接续一个艾炷。

During moxibustion, a moxa cone of about 10mm in bottom diameter and about 15mm in height is placed on the ginger slices, and the moxa cone is ignited from the top, followed by another moxa cone thereon when the former is being finished.

灰烬过多时及时清理。

When there is too much ash, it should be cleaned up in time.

注意艾灸过程中要不断地移动姜片,以局部出现大片红晕,患者觉温热为度。

It should be noted that, in the process of moxibustion, the ginger slices should be constantly moved to the extent that they make a large area flush and make patients feel a little bit warm.

常用于呕吐、泻痢、腹痛、肾虚遗精、风寒湿痹、面瘫、麻木酸痛、肢体痿软无力等病症（见图 2-14）。

Ginger moxibustion is commonly used to treat vomiting, diarrhea, abdominal pain, emission with deficiency of the kidney, wind-cold-dampness arthralgia, facial paralysis, numbness and aching pain, flaccid paralysis and asthenia of limbs and other diseases (see Fig. 2-14).

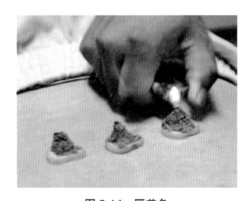

图 2-14　隔姜灸
Fig. 2-14　Ginger moxibustion

2. 隔蒜灸　取独头大蒜切成 2~3mm 的蒜片，在其上用针点刺小孔若干。

2. Garlic Moxibustion　A one-clove garlic is cut into slices of 2-3mm in thickness, on which quick puncture is performed with a needle, forming several tiny holes.

施灸时，将一底面直径约 10mm、高约 15mm 的圆锥形艾炷放置蒜片上，从顶端点燃艾炷，待快燃烧尽时在上面接续一个艾炷。

During moxibustion, a moxa cone of about 10mm in bottom diameter and about 15mm in height is placed on the garlic slices, and the moxa cone is ignited from the top, followed by another moxa cone thereon when the former is being finished.

灰烬过多时及时清理。

When there is too much ash, it should be cleaned up in time.

注意艾灸过程中要不断地移动蒜片，以局部出现大片红晕潮湿，患者觉热为度。

It should be noted that, in the process of moxibustion, the garlic slices should be constantly moved to the extent that they make a large area flush and wet and make patients feel hot.

常用于阴疽流注、疮色发白,不红不痛,不化脓者。

Garlic moxibustion is commonly used for the patients suffering from deep multiple abscess with white skin and without flush and pain as well as fester.

对疔疮疖毒、乳痈等急性炎症,未溃者也可灸之。

It can also be used for the patients suffering from sores and furuncles, mammary carbuncles and other acute inflammations without fester.

也可用于治疗虫、蛇咬伤和蜂蝎蜇伤或无名肿毒。

It can also be used in the treatment of insect bites, snake bites, wasp and scorpion stings or unnamed toxic swelling.

3. **隔盐灸** 一般用于神阙穴灸,用食盐填平脐孔,上放底面直径约 10mm、高约 15mm 的圆锥形艾炷,从顶端点燃艾炷,待快燃烧尽时再接续一个艾炷。

3. Salt Moxibustion It is commonly used for the moxibustion of Shenque point, for which the umbilicus should be filled with salt, and then a moxa cone of about 10mm in bottom diameter and about 15mm in height is placed on the salt. The moxa cone is ignited from the top, followed by another moxa cone thereon when the former is being finished.

灰烬过多时及时清理,以腹腔觉热为度。

When there is too much ash, it should be cleaned up in time. The therapy should be finished to the extent that the abdominal cavity feels hot.

常用于霍乱吐泻致肢冷脉伏者,以及寒证腹痛、虚寒性痢疾、中风脱证的四肢厥冷及虚脱休克等,可有急救之效。

It is commonly used for the patients with cold limbs and hidden pulse due to vomiting and diarrhea, abdominal pain due to cold, diarrhea due to deficiency and coldness, cold limbs and torpid shock due to apoplectic collapse, etc. It can be used as an emergency treatment.

4. **隔附子饼灸** 用附子研成细粉,加白及粉或面粉少许,再用水调和捏成薄饼,底面直径约 20mm,厚度 2~5mm,待稍干用针刺小孔若干。

4. Monkshood Cake Moxibustion　Monkshood is pulverized into fine powder with the addition of common bletilla rubber powder or a little bit of flour, mixed with water and kneaded into thin cakes, which are about 20mm in bottom diameter and about 2-5mm in thickness and are punctured with a needle, forming several tiny holes when they are a little bit dry.

施灸时,将一底面直径约10mm、高约15mm的圆锥形艾炷放置药饼上,从顶端点燃艾炷,待快燃烧尽时在上面接续一个艾炷,灰烬过多应及时清理。

During moxibustion, a moxa cone of about 10mm in bottom diameter and about 15mm in height is placed on the medicated cake, and the moxa cone is ignited from the top, followed by another moxa cone thereon when the former is being finished. When there is too much ash, it should be cleaned up in time.

一饼灸干再换一饼,以患者觉微微烘热为度。

When finished, a cake should be replaced with another one, and the therapy should be finished to the extent that patients feel a little bit warm.

常用于虚寒性病症及外科术后疮疡溃后久不收口者,其可祛腐生肌、促使愈合(见图2-15)。

It is commonly used in the treatment of diseases resulting from deficiency and coldness, and slow-healing of swelling and ulceration following surgery. The therapy can remove the necrotic tissue and promote granulation for healing (see Fig.2-15).

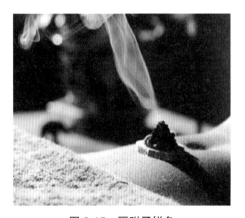

图 2-15　隔附子饼灸
Fig.2-15　Monkshood cake moxibustion

二、临床应用

Ⅱ. Clinical Application

（一）适用范围

（Ⅰ）Scope of Application

隔物灸由于使用的介质不同,因而产生的治疗功效亦有所区别,隔物灸通过对穴位的持续温灸,对人体的风湿骨病、神经内科疾病、内分泌系统疾病、免疫系统疾病、消化系统疾病、呼吸系统疾病、循环系统疾病、泌尿生殖系统疾病等均有显著疗效。

Indirect moxibustion has different therapeutic effects due to the use of different medium. Through the continuous warm moxibustion of acupoints, it has obvious therapeutic effects on rheumatoid bone diseases, neurological diseases, endocrine system diseases, immune system diseases, digestive system diseases, respiratory diseases, circulatory system diseases, genitourinary system diseases, etc.

（二）处方示例

（Ⅱ）Prescription Examples

1. **面瘫病（周围性面瘫）** 面瘫常由风寒外袭,入中面部经络,以一侧面部肌肉瘫痪、额纹消失、眼裂变大、露睛流泪、鼻唇沟变浅、口角㖞向健侧为主要临床表现,部分患者初起时有耳后疼痛。

1. **Facial Paralysis（Peripheral Facial Paralysis）** Facial paralysis commonly results from invasion of the facial meridians and collaterals by cold-wind pathogens, which is clinically characterized by paralysis of the muscles of one side of the face, disappearance of the wrinkles on the forehead, enlargement of palpebral fissure, lacrimation with eyes half-closed, shallowing of the nasolabial groove, and the corner of the mouth tilting to the healthy side, and some patients initially suffer from the pain in the postauricular part.

治法:温经通络。
Treatment Method: Warming meridians and dredging collaterals.

灸法:隔姜灸。
Moxibustion Method: Ginger moxibustion.

操作：选用患侧阳白、下关、颊车、地仓、颧髎等穴，每穴灸 3~4 壮，或以局部红晕、觉微微烘热为度。

Operation：3-4 moxa cones are used for each of Yangbai，Xiaguan，Jiache，Dicang，Quanliao，etc. on the affected side，which should flush locally and feel warm.

每日或隔日 1 次，5~7 次为 1 个疗程。

It should be performed once daily or every other day，and 5-7 times constitute a course of treatment.

灸后避风寒。

After moxibustion，wind-cold should be avoided.

2. 鼻鼽（变应性鼻炎） 本病多由肺气虚弱，脾肾虚损，卫表不固，腠理疏松，风寒湿邪乘虚而入，邪气相搏，肺气不宣，侵犯鼻窍所致。

2. Allergic Rhinitis（Anaphylactic Rhinitis） This disease is resulting from obstruction of lung qi invading nasal orifices，which is mainly caused by insufficiency of lung qi，impairment of the spleen and kidney，failure of defensive qi to protect the body，looseness of the striae of the skin and muscles and thus pathogenic wind，cold and dampness invade the body by taking advantage of weak body resistance.

临床主要表现为喷嚏、鼻塞、鼻痒、流涕等。

The main clinical manifestations include sneezing，nasal congestion，rhinocnesmus，watery nasal discharge，etc.

治法：扶阳补气。
Treatment Method：Strengthening yang and tonifying qi.

灸法：隔姜灸。
Moxibustion Method：Ginger moxibustion.

操作：选用上印堂、风门、肺俞、大椎等穴，每穴 3~5 壮，以局部红晕、温热为度。

Operation：3-5 moxa cones are used for each of Yintang，Fengmen，Feishu，Dazhui and other acupoints，which should flush locally and feel warm.

每日 1 次, 10 次为 1 个疗程。

It should be performed once daily and 10 times constitute a course of treatment.

灸后避风寒。

After moxibustion, wind-cold should be avoided.

3. 咳嗽（急慢性支气管炎） 咳嗽是因邪客肺系, 肺失宣肃, 肺气不清所致, 以咳嗽、咳痰为主要症状的病症。

3. Cough（Acute or Chronic Bronchitis） Cough results from failure of lung qi to disperse and purify caused by invasion of pathogens into the lung system, with the main symptoms of cough and expectoration.

分为外感咳嗽和内伤咳嗽, 外感咳嗽多由外邪侵袭而引起, 内伤咳嗽为脏腑功能失调所致。

It falls into exogenous cough and endogenous cough. The former mostly results from invasion of exogenous pathogenic factors and the latter results from dysfunctional zang-fu organs.

治法:温肺止咳、补虚固本。

Treatment Method: Warming the lung to relieve cough and tonifying deficiency to consolidate the constitution.

灸法:隔姜灸。

Moxibustion Method: Ginger moxibustion.

操作:选取肺俞、膏肓、足三里、肾俞等穴, 每穴 5 壮, 以局部红晕、温热为度。

Operation: 5 moxa cones are used for each of Feishu, Gaohuang, Zusanli, Shenshu and other acupoints, which should flush locally and feel warm.

每日或隔日 1 次, 5~7 次为 1 个疗程。

It should be performed once daily or every other day, and 5-7 times constitute a course of treatment.

灸后避风寒。

After moxibustion, wind-cold should be avoided.

4. 哮病（支气管哮喘） 本病多为阳气虚弱、肺脾肾虚、痰饮留伏所致。

4. Asthma（Bronchial Asthma） This disease comes from yang qi deficiency, insufficiency of the lung, spleen and kidney, and retention of phlegm and fluid.

病属阴属寒，且易在冬季发作。

This disease is of yin and cold properties and mostly occurs in winter.

该病可因外邪侵袭、饮食不当、情志刺激、身体劳倦等引发，以致痰壅气道、肺气宣降功能失常而发病。

This disease may occur under the conditions of phlegm retention in the airway with dysfunction of lung qi in dispersion and purification, which is mostly caused by invasion of exogenous pathogenic factors, improper diet, emotional stimulation and fatigue.

发作时临床表现可有喉间痰鸣、气促、呼吸困难，甚则喘息不能平卧，痰多清稀或黄稠而黏。

When breaking out, the disease clinically manifests itself as wheezing with retention of phlegm in throat, shortness of breath, dyspnea, even failure to lie flat due to dyspnea, copious watery phlegm or yellow, thick and sticky phlegm.

缓解期可无症状或仅咳嗽、胸闷等症状。

In remission stage, it may be asymptomatic or manifests itself as only cough, chest tightness, etc.

治法：温肺止喘、补虚固本。

Treatment Method: Warming the lung to relieve asthma and tonifying deficiency to consolidate the constitution.

灸法：隔姜灸、隔附子饼灸。

Moxibustion Method: Ginger moxibustion and monkshood cake moxibustion.

操作：选取大椎、风门、肺俞、定喘等穴隔姜灸，每穴 5~7 壮，或以局部红晕、温热为度。

Operation: The ginger moxibustion is performed on each of Dazhui, Fengmen, Feishu, Dingchuan and other acupoints, for which 5-7 cones should be used, or which should flush locally and feel warm.

每日或隔日 1 次,10 次为 1 个疗程。

It should be performed once daily or every other day, and 10 times constitute a course of treatment.

灸后避风寒。

After moxibustion, wind-cold should be avoided.

5. 痛经(原发性痛经)　痛经多由寒凝胞中、气滞血瘀所致。

5. Dysmenorrhea(Primary Dysmenorrhea)　Dysmenorrhea is mostly caused by cold congealing in the uterus and Qi-stagnation and blood stasis.

临床表现为从月经初潮开始,行经前后或月经期出现下腹疼痛、坠胀,经色紫暗、夹有瘀块,伴腰酸或其他不适症状如头痛、乏力、头晕、恶心、呕吐等,但生殖器官无器质性病变。

It clinically manifests itself as lower abdominal pain, tenesmus and distention, dark menses with blood mass, accompanied by sore waist or other uncomfortable symptoms such as headache, fatigue, dizziness, nausea, vomiting, etc. The disease may occur from menarche, before and after menstruation or during menstrual period, without organic lesions in the reproductive organs.

治法:温经散寒,祛瘀止痛。

Treatment Method:Warming meridian and dispersing cold, and removing stasis to ease pain.

灸法:隔盐灸、隔姜灸。

Moxibustion Method:Salt moxibustion and ginger moxibustion.

操作:神阙穴隔盐灸,先将纯净干燥食盐填于神阙穴中,使之与脐平,然后上置大艾炷点燃施灸,当艾炷燃尽后,易炷再灸,直至规定壮数。

Operation:Shenque point salt moxibustion, pure dry salt should be first filled in Shenque point, flush with the umbilicus. Then a large moxa cone should be placed and ignited for moxibustion, and when burning away, the moxa cone should be replaced with another one up to the specified number of moxa cones.

关元、水道、归来等穴用隔姜灸。

Ginger moxibustion should be used for Guanyuan, Shuidao, Guilai, etc.

施灸中若患者感觉灼热疼痛不能忍受时,可用镊子上下移动姜片,切勿烫伤。

If patients feel unbearably burning and painful during moxibustion, the ginger slices should be moved up and down to prevent burning by using tweezers.

轻度痛经每次灸 4 壮,中度 6 壮,重度 8 壮。

4 moxa cones can be used for mild dysmenorrhea at a time, 6 moxa cones for moderate case and 8 moxa cones for severe case.

可在月经周期经前 2~3 天开始施灸,每天 1 次,3~5 次为 1 疗程(月经周期),共治疗 3 个疗程。

2-3 days before the menstrual cycle, moxibustion can be performed once a day, and 3-5 times constitute a course of treatment (menstrual cycle), with 3 courses of treatment in total.

6. 疖 疖是指肌肤浅表部位感受火毒,致局部红肿热痛为主要表现的急性化脓性疾病,包括有头疖、无头疖、疖病。

6. Furuncles Furuncles refer to the acute suppurative disease which is caused by invasion of the superficial part of the body by fire toxin. It mainly shows local redness, swelling, hotness and pain, and it includes headed furuncle, headless furuncle and furunculosis.

治法:祛邪排毒。

Treatment Method: Eliminating of pathogen and toxin.

灸法:隔蒜灸。

Moxibustion Method: Garlic moxibustion.

操作:在疮疖中心隔蒜灸,每穴 5~7 壮,或以疖周潮红、温热为度。

Operation: Garlic moxibustion is performed on the centers of the sores and furuncles, for each of which 5 to 7 moxa cones should be used, or the furuncles should flush around and feel warm.

每日 1 次,3 次为 1 个疗程。

It should be performed once daily, and 3 times constitute a course of treatment.

三、禁忌证

Ⅲ. Contraindications

1. 糖尿病或其他疾病等引起感觉功能减退、皮肤愈合能力差者忌用。

1. It is contraindicated for the patients who suffer from diabetes or those diseases with sensory dysfunction and poor skin healing ability.

2. 小儿皮肤娇嫩,不宜灸。

2. Children's skin is delicate and not suitable for moxibustion.

孕妇不宜使用,防止坠胎或早产。

It is contraindicated for pregnant women lest abortion or premature delivery.

四、注意事项

Ⅳ. Precautions

1. 隔物灸操作过程中应注意勤动勤看,以防起疱。

1. In the process of indirect moxibustion, frequent attention should be paid to preventing blisters.

2. 穴位处有皮损、皮疹、溃疡者禁用。

2. It is contraindicated for the patients with skin lesions, rashes and ulcers.

3. 施灸期间勿洗冷水澡,切勿过劳。

3. During moxibustion, cold showers and overfatigue are prohibited.

除个别疼痛较重对症治疗外,其余不配用其他治疗方法。

Except that the individual patients with more severe pain should be treated accordingly, no one needs related therapy.

4. 久咳肺虚及阴虚火旺者忌用。

4. It is contraindicated for the patients with chronic cough due to lung deficiency and hyperactive fire from yin deficiency.

对皮肤黏膜有刺激,易发疱,皮肤过敏者忌用。

It is contraindicated for the patients with skin mucosa susceptible to irritation,blisters and allergies.

五、意外情况处理方法

V. Treatment for Accidents

1. 在施灸过程中若不慎灼伤皮肤,致皮肤起水疱,须注意防止感染。

1. In the process of moxibustion,in case that the skin is accidentally burned to develop blisters,attention must be paid to preventing infection.

2. 偶尔出现过敏者,可擦抗过敏药膏,并戒食鱼虾、生鸡蛋等易致敏的食物,必要时医院就诊。

2. Occasionally there may come patients who are allergic,then the anti-allergy ointment can be used for them,and they should abstain from taking in fishes and shrimps,raw eggs and other foods that easily induce allergy. They should go to hospital if necessary.

参 考 文 献

References

[1] 徐家淳,李岩,赵祥斐,等.浅谈灸法禁忌的历史沿革[J].中华针灸电子杂志,2013,2 (5):238-240.

[2] 赵亮,卢建华,周凤玲.中国传统文化对现代医学技术创新的影响[J].中国西部科技, 2011,10(21):45-47.

[3] 谢华,易受乡,易展,等.灸法量效关系的研究进展与思考[J].中华中医药学刊,2010, 28(5):1003-1005.

[4] 李西忠,李忠正,席强,等.影响灸法作用因素的研究进展[J].针灸临床杂志,2008,26 (8):58-61,69.

[5] 傅小苏.近年来灸法作用机理的研究进展及临床应用[J].针灸临床杂志,2003(3): 52-53,59.

[6] 马彦红.浅谈《内经》灸法[J].河北中医,2004,26(1):48.

第四节 温 针 灸

Section 4 Warming Needle Moxibustion

温针灸法,又称"温针""针柄灸"及"烧针柄"等,是利用艾条段或艾炷固定在毫针针柄施灸,将艾灸和针刺结合在一起使用的治疗技术。

Warming needle moxibustion, also called "warming needle acupuncture", "needle handle moxibustion" or "burning needle handle", is a therapy which fixes moxa sticks or moxa cones onto the handles of filiform needles to give moxibustion and uses the moxibustion and acupuncture together.

温针之名首见于《伤寒论》,但其方法不详。

The name of the warming needle first appears in the *Treatise on Cold Pathogenic Diseases*, but its methods are unknown.

明代高武的《针灸聚英》及杨继洲的《针灸大成》均有施灸方法的记载。

The warming needle moxibustion is recorded both in *An Exemplary Collection of Acupuncture and Moxibustion and their Essentials* by Gao Wu, and the *Compendium of Acupuncture and Moxibustion* by Yang Jizhou in Ming Dynasty.

温针灸的治疗机制主要是针刺的作用、艾灸的温热效应和针体的导热效应综合叠加的效果。

The therapy mechanism is mainly the comprehensive effect of the function of acupuncture, warming effect of moxibustion and heat conduction effect of needle body.

本法多用于风湿等偏于寒性疾病的治疗。

The therapy is mainly used for treating diseases of cold nature such as rheumatism.

一、温针灸操作技术

I. Operating Techniques of Warming Needle Moxibustion

温针灸是将灸法与刺法相联合的一种治疗方式,把针刺和灸法的优点相结合,使艾灸产生的热能通过针体深入穴位,通过调理脏腑经络,促进机体的新陈代谢,增强人体的免疫功能,从而具备防病治病的疗效。

The warming needle moxibustion is a therapy combining moxibustion and acupuncture, and especially their advantages to make the heat energy generated by moxibustion deeply embedded in acupoints through the needle, promoting body's metabolism by conditioning zang-fu organs, meridians and collaterals and improving the immune function of human body, thereby having therapeutic effects of preventing and curing diseases.

(一) 灸前准备

(Ⅰ) Preparation

1. 针具选择　应选长柄针,一般在 28 号以下最好,长短适度,刺在肌肉深厚处。

1. Selection of Needles　A needle with a longer handle should be selected, usually the needle being larger No. 28, with a suitable length to puncture into the acupoints with thicker muscles.

2. 艾绒放置　将艾炷或艾绒搓团捻裹于针柄上点燃,通过针体将热力传入穴位。

2. Position of Moxa wool　The moxa cone or moxa wool being rolled into a wick is twisted and wrapped onto the handle, and then is ignited. The heating power is transmitted to the acupoints through the needle body.

每次燃烧枣核大艾团或艾炷 1~3 壮。

Every time a moxa ball with the size of a date pit or 1-3 zhuangs of moxa cones are burned.

3. 穴位选择　温针灸主要刺激区为体穴、阿是穴。

3. Selection of Acupoints　The body acupoints and Ashi points are mainly selected for the warming needle moxibustion.

(二) 施灸方法

Ⅱ. Methods of Moxibustion

先取长度在 1.5 寸以上的毫针,刺入穴位得气后,留针不动,针柄与表皮相距 2~3 分为宜。

The filiform needle with a length of 1.5 cun or more is firstly penetrated into the acupoints, and after arrival of qi, the needle is retained, with a suitable distance of 2-3 fen between the handle of needle and the skin.

将硬纸片剪成方寸块,中钻一孔,从针柄上套入,以保护穴位周围之皮肤,防止落下火团烧伤,在留针过程中,于针柄上裹以纯艾绒的艾团,或取 2cm 长艾条一段,套在针柄之上,无论艾团、艾条段均应距皮肤 2~3cm,再从其下端用线香点燃施灸(见图 2-16)。

A piece of hard paper is cut into a block with one inch square, a hole is drilled at the middle of the block, and the block is sheathed from the handle for protecting the skin around the acupoints, and preventing the fire ball falling off to burn the skin. In the process of retaining the needle, a pure moxa ball is wrapped onto the handle, or the section of the moxa stick with a length of 2cm is selected, and is sheathed onto the handle. The moxa balls and sticks both should have a 2-3cm distance from the skin, and then should be ignited from the ends by incense stick to conduct moxibustion (see Fig.2-16).

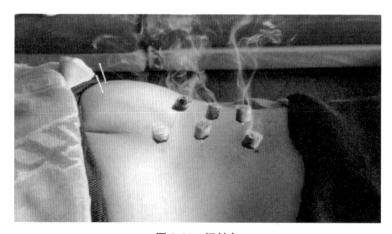

图 2-16 温针灸
Fig. 2-16 Warming needle moxibustion

施灸中如果过热,可将毫针向上提一些,以觉温热而不灼痛为度。

During moxibustion, if the needle is overheated, the filiform needle can be raised upward, to achieve the effect of feeling warm rather than causalgic.

每次如果用艾团可灸 3~4 壮,艾条段则只需 1~2 壮。

Every time, 3-4 zhuangs of moxa wool should be chosen in the size of moxa ball, and 1-2 zhuangs in the size of moxa stick.

近年,还采用帽状艾炷进行温针灸。

In recent years, the cap-shaped moxa cone is also used for warming needle moxibustion.

帽状艾炷主要成分为艾叶炭,类似无烟艾条,但其长度为2cm,直径1cm,一端有小孔,点燃后可插于针柄上,燃烧时间为30分钟。

The main component of the cap-shaped moxa cone is charred argy wormwood leaves, being similar to smokeless moxa stick. However it is 2cm in length, and 1cm in diameter, with a small hole in one end. After being ignited, the moxa cone can be inserted into the handle, and the burning time is 30 minutes.

因其外形像小帽,可戴于毫针上,又称帽炷灸。

Because its shape is like a cap, the moxa cone can be worn on the filiform needle, and is also called cap-shaped moxa-cone moxibustion.

帽炷温针灸,既无烟,也不会污染空气,同时作用时间又长,是一种较为理想的温针灸法。

The cap-shaped moxa-cone warming needle moxibustion is a comparatively ideal warming needle moxibustion which is smokeless, cannot pollute air, and at the same time has a long action time.

二、临床应用

II. Clinical Application

(一)适用范围
(I) Scope of Application

本灸法可用于治疗风寒湿痹、骨质增生、腰腿痛、关节酸痛、冠心病、高脂血症、痛风、胃脘痛、腹痛、腹泻等。

The moxibustion is used for treating wind-cold-damp impediment, hyperosteogeny, pain in the waist and lower extremities, joint pain, coronary artery heart disease, hyperlipemia, gout, gastralgia, abdominal pain, diarrhea, etc.

（二）处方示例

（Ⅱ）Prescription Examples

1. 项痹病（神经根型颈椎病）　本病常因督脉劳损、气血不足、感受外邪等导致经脉闭阻，以颈项部疼痛及上肢麻木，头、颈、肩部活动受限，甚者影响日常工作和生活为主要表现。

1. Nape Impediment（Cervical Spondylotic Radiculopathy）　The disease is resulting from obstruction of meridians, usually caused by strain of the Du meridian, deficiency of qi and blood, invasion of exogenous pathogens, etc. The major manifestations are pain in the neck and napex, numbness of upper limbs, limitation of action of the head, neck and shoulders, and even influence daily work and life.

治法：舒筋活血、通络止痛、松解粘连、滑利关节。

Treatment Methods：Relieving rigidity of muscles and promoting blood circulation, dredging collaterals to stop pain, releasing adhesion and lubricating joints.

处方：颈夹脊、阿是穴、天柱穴、后溪穴、申脉穴。

Acupoints：Jingjiaji, Ashi points, Tianzhu, Houxi and Shenmai.

体位：患者仰卧位，医者站于患者右侧，检查患者头部前屈、后伸及向左右旋转活动度并进行记录。

Position：The patient should be in supine position, and the doctor stands at the right side of the patient to examine the ranges of the patient's head movements in anteflexion, retro-extension, levorotation and dextrorotation, and then records their moving situation.

点燃灸炷：待施针结束后，点燃针尾的艾炷，待其自行燃尽。

Ignition of Moxibustion Cone：After the needling is over, the moxa cone located on the end of the needle is ignited to burn itself out.

检查患侧的活动度并与治疗前进行比较。

The range of motion of the affected side is examined and is compared with that before the treatment.

如果病情没有改善，继续调整针刺深度至临床症状改善。

If the patient's condition is not improved, the acupuncture depth is continually adjusted to achieve the improvement of the clinical symptoms.

特别提示:

Special notes:

①在针刺过程中用双手托住患者枕部,引导向运动障碍方向做徐缓的主动运动。

①During the process of acupuncture, the patient's occiput is held with both hands, to guide the occiput towards the dyskinesia direction to make slowly active movement.

②症状较轻者,在针刺过程中即可进行适当的颈部前屈后伸、左右侧屈及环转等主动运动。

②During the process of acupuncture, the patient with mild symptoms can make appropriate active movements on the neck such as anteflexion and retro-extension, levo-lateral flexion, dextro-lateral flexion circle rotation, etc.

2. 肩凝症(肩关节周围炎) 本病主要是因为外伤劳损,筋脉失养;

2. Frozen Shoulder(Periarthritis of Shoulder Joints) This disease is mainly caused by trauma, strain, or malnutrition of the tendons and meridians;

或肝肾阴虚,气血不足,不能濡养筋骨;

or yin deficiency of the liver and kidney, and deficiency of qi and blood, with malnutrition of the tendons and bones;

或外感风寒湿邪,脉络拘急所致,主要表现为肩部疼痛和功能障碍。

or invasion by exogenous wind-cold-dampness pathogens. It is mainly manifested as shoulder pain and functional disturbance.

治法:舒筋活血、通络止痛、松解粘连、滑利关节。

Treatment Methods: Relieving rigidity of muscles and promoting blood circulation, dredging collaterals to stop pain, releasing adhesion and lubricating joints.

处方:鱼际、外关、阳陵泉、听宫、养老。

Acupoints: Yuji, Waiguan, Yanglingquan, Tinggong and Yanglao.

体位:患者仰卧位,医者站于患者右侧,检查患肢的外展、外旋被动活动度并进行记录。

Position:The patient should be in supine position, and the doctor stands at the right side of the patient to examine the ranges of movements of the affected limb in abduction and extorsion, and then records their moving situation.

点燃灸炷:待施针结束后,点燃针尾的艾炷,待其自行燃尽。

Ignition of Moxibustion Cone:After the needling is over, the moxa cone located on the end of the needle is ignited to burn itself out.

检查患肢的外展、外旋被动活动度并与治疗前进行比较。

Examine the ranges of passive movements of abduction and extorsion of the affected limb, and compare with those prior to treatment.

如果病情没有改善,继续调整针刺深度至临床症状改善。

If the patient's condition is not improved, the acupuncture depth is continually adjusted to achieve the improvement of the clinical symptoms.

特别提示:

Special Notes:

在治疗同时必须配合适当的肩部功能锻炼,要求患者持之以恒,循序渐进,因人而异。

The appropriate shoulder function exercise must be added in treatment. The patient must persevere and must follow in order and advance step by step, of course, it varies from person to person.

方法可选用前后摆动、回旋运动、爬墙高举、内收外展及牵拉滑车等。

The useful methods include forward and backward swing, rotation, wall climbing and lifting, adduction and abduction, pulley traction, etc.

3. 膝痹病(膝关节骨性关节炎) 本病常因膝关节周围软组织慢性劳损、肝肾不足、外邪闭阻经脉所致。

3. Knee Impediment(Knee Osteoarthritis) This disease is often caused by soft tissue chronic strain surrounding knee joint, insufficiency of liver and kidney, and invasion of exogenous pathogens into the meridians.

临床以膝关节疼痛、肿胀、活动受限为主要表现。

It is mainly manifested as knee joint pain, swelling and limited movement.

活动或天气变化时疼痛加重,常反复发作。

Pain becomes severer during movement or weather change, and usually repeatedly occurs.

治法:舒筋活血、通络止痛、松解粘连、滑利关节。

Treatment Methods: Relieving rigidity of muscles and promoting blood circulation, dredging meridians to stop pain, releasing adhesion and lubricating joints.

处方:梁丘、血海、内膝眼、外膝眼、阴陵泉、阳陵泉。

Acupoints: Liangqiu, Xuehai, Neixiyan (EX-LE4), Waixiyan (Dubi), Yinlingquan and Yanglingquan.

体位:患者仰卧位,医者站于患者右侧,检查患膝的屈伸活动度并进行记录。

Position: The patient should be in supine position, and the doctor stands at the right side of the patient to examine the ranges of bending of the patient's affected knee, and records its moving situation.

点燃灸炷:待施针结束后,点燃针尾的艾炷,待其自行燃尽。

Ignition of moxibustion cone: After the needling is over, the moxa cone located on the end of the needle is ignited to burn itself out.

检查患膝的活动度并与治疗前进行比较。

The ranges of movement of the affected knee are examined and compared with that before the treatment.

如果病情没有改善,继续调整针刺深度至临床症状改善。

If the patient's condition is not improved, the acupuncture depth is continually adjusted to achieve the improvement of the clinical symptoms.

三、禁忌证

Ⅲ. Contraindication

1. 凝血功能障碍的患者禁用。

1. It is prohibited for the patients with blood coagulation disorders.

2. 孕妇禁用。

2. It is prohibited for pregnant women.

3. 皮肤感觉迟钝及小儿患者禁用。

3. It is prohibited for the patients with hypaesthesia and pediatric patients.

4. 极度疲劳、过饥、过饱、酒醉、高热及无自控能力的患者禁用。

4. It is prohibited for the patients with exhaustion, polyorexia, hyperhagia, drunkenness and hyperpyrexia and without self-control ability.

四、注意事项

Ⅳ. Precautions

1. 医生要在平时反复练习缠绕艾炷的手法,熟练者一触即妥,几秒钟就能牢固地放在针柄上。

1. The doctors should repeatedly practice the technique of winding the moxa cone. Skilled doctors can firmly put the moxa cone on the needle in a few seconds.

2. 温针灸的艾炷要光圆紧实,切忌松散,以防脱落。

2. The moxa cone for the warming needle moxibustion should be smooth, round and tight, should not be loose, so as to prevent falling off.

3. 温针灸要严防艾火脱落烧灼皮肤。

3. Pay more attention to moxa fire to prevent its falling off to burn the skin during this therapy.

可预先用硬纸剪成圆形纸片,并剪一位于中心的小缺口,置于针下穴位上。

Λ piece of hard paper may be cut into small round pieces in advance, with a small notch in the center. One piece is put onto the acupoint under the needle.

4. 温针灸时,要嘱咐患者不要随意移动肢体,以防灼伤。

4. In the process of warming needle moxibustion, the patients should be asked not to randomly move limbs so as to prevent burning.

五、意外情况处理方法

V. Treatment for Accidents

1. 在施灸过程中,若万一不慎灼伤皮肤,致皮肤起透明发亮的水疱,须注意防止感染。

1. In the process of moxibustion, in case the skin is accidentally burned to the extent that transparent and bright blisters form, attention must be paid to preventing infection.

2. 该方法简便易行,但是要注意防止因针尾烧灼过热而折针。

2. The therapy is simple and convenient, but attention must be paid to prevent needle breakage due to cauterization of the end of the needle.

参 考 文 献

References

[1] 王富春. 刺法灸法学[M]. 上海:上海科学技术出版社,2009:57.

[2] 冯淑兰. 刺法灸法学[M]. 北京:科学技术文献出版社,2006:84.

[3] 赵吉平,李俊. 灸法、拔罐与刮痧法入门[M]. 北京:人民卫生出版社,2008:41.

[4] 陶晓雁,殷仕洁,毛湄,等. 从近10年灸法文献看灸法的特色与优势[J]. 辽宁中医杂志,2008,12(4):591-593.

[5] 常小荣,严洁,王超,等. 灸法的历史沿革及前景展望[J]. 中华中医药学刊,2008(7):1433-1435.

[6] 吴焕淦,刘立公,陈跃来,等. 灸法的继承与创新[J]. 上海针灸杂志,2007(12):39-41.

第五节 督 灸

Section 5 Du Moxibustion

督灸,又称长蛇灸,是指于督脉的脊柱段施以"隔姜泥铺灸",属于传统艾灸疗法中的一种,督灸通过激发协调诸经,发挥平衡阴阳、抵御病邪、调整虚实的功效,从而达到预防保健的目的。

Du moxibustion, also called long snake moxibustion, refers to moxibustion of applying "Ginger-Spreading Moxibustion" to the spinal segment of Du meridian. It belongs to one of the traditional moxibustion therapies. By stimulating and coordinating various meridians to perform functions of balancing yin and yang, resisting pathogenic factors and adjusting deficiency and excess, Du moxibustion achieves the purposes of prevention and health care.

督灸基本作用包括:调节免疫功能,调节神经 - 内分泌功能,抗自由基、抗氧化等。

Du moxibustion has the basic functions: Adjusting immunity, adjusting nerve and endocrine, resisting free radicals, resisting oxidation and the like.

中医学认为,阳气为人体之本,阳气对脏腑有温煦推动的作用,阳气的虚弱与不足会导致多种疾病,而督脉是"阳脉之海",位于人体正中后脊,总督诸阳。

TCM holds that yang qi is the foundation of a human body, yang qi has the effects of warming and invigorating the zang-fu organs, the deficiency and insufficiency of yang qi may lead to various diseases, and Du meridian, as "the sea of yang meridians", is situated in the median backbone of the human body and controls all yang meridians generally.

督灸通过强壮真元、调和阴阳、温通气血的方法治疗疾病。

Therefore, Du moxibustion can treat diseases by strengthening genuine qi, regulating yin and yang, and warming qi and blood.

该疗法取穴多用大椎穴至腰俞穴间督脉段,是目前灸疗中施灸范围最大,一次治疗时间最长的灸法(见图 2-17)。

This therapy mainly selects the Du meridian segment from Dazhui point to Yaoshu point. It is a therapy with a widest moxibustion scope and longest treatment course at present(see Fig. 2-17).

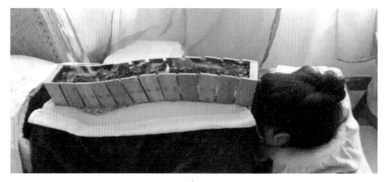

图 2-17 督灸
Fig. 2-17 Du moxibustion

一、督灸操作技术

I. Operating Technology of Du Moxibustion

督灸通过在督脉的脊柱段上施以治疗,将经络、腧穴、药物、艾灸的综合作用融为一体,充分发挥温肾壮阳、行气破瘀、拔毒散结、祛寒利湿、通督止痛的功效,以达益肾通督、温阳散寒、壮骨透肌、破瘀散结、通痹止痛的治疗作用,具有治疗时间长、作用持久、疗效可靠,且安全无副作用的特点。

By performing treatment on the spinal column segment of Du meridian, Du moxibustion integrates combined functions of meridians, collaterals, acupoints, medicine and moxibustion, gives full play to the actions of warming the kidney to invigorate yang, activating qi and removing blood stasis, draining toxin and dissipating nodulation, dispelling cold and removing dampness, dredging Du meridian to stop pain, so as to achieve the treatment effects of tonifying the kidney and dredging Du meridian, warming yang to dispel cold, strengthening bone and reinforcing muscles, drastically removing blood stasis and lump, and removing obstruction to stop pain. It is characterized by a longer course of treatment, a lasting action, reliable curative effect, safety and no side effect.

(一)灸前准备

(I) Preparation Before Moxibustion

督灸操作时需要准备艾绒、生姜 1 000g、督灸灸具、督灸粉、打火机、镊子、酒精棉球、无菌纱布、刮痧板、刮痧油。

Before Du moxibustion operation, it is required to prepare moxa wool, fresh ginger of 1 000g, moxibustion implement, moxibustion powder, cigarette lighter, tweezers, alcohol cotton ball, sterile gauze, scraping board and scraping oil.

（二）施灸方法

（Ⅱ）Methods for Moxibustion

1. 施灸部位　取督脉的大椎穴至腰俞穴为施灸部位。

1. Moxibustion part　From Dazhui point to Yaoshu point of Du meridian.

2. 施灸程序

2. Moxibustion Procedure

（1）病人取俯卧位，使全身放松，暴露治疗部位。

（1）Let the patient take a prone position, relax the whole body and expose the treatment area.

（2）取穴：取督脉的大椎穴至腰俞穴为施灸部位。

（2）Selecting acupoints：Select the segment from Dazhui point to Yaoshu point of Du meridian as the moxibustion part.

（3）刮痧：沿着背部督脉、膀胱经进行刮痧，帮助疏通经络。

（3）Scrapping：Perform scrapping along Du meridian and bladder meridian to help dredge meridians and collaterals.

（4）消毒：以酒精棉球沿施术部位自上而下常规消毒 3 遍。

（4）Sterilization：Perform routine sterilization for three times from top to bottom along the moxibustion part with alcohol cotton ball.

（5）撒督灸粉：在治疗部位薄撒一层督灸粉，之后在其上覆盖无菌纱布。

（5）Scattering moxibustion powder：Scatter a layer of moxibustion powder on the treatment area, and then put sterile gauze thereon.

（6）铺姜泥：将姜泥平铺于无菌纱布上，要求上下均匀，薄厚一致，约 1.5cm。

（6）Spreading ginger paste：Spread ginger paste on the sterile gauze uniformly from top to bottom with uniform thickness of about 1.5cm.

（7）放置灸具：在灸具底部薄铺一层姜泥，并放置于施灸部位上。

（7）Placing moxibustion implement：Spread a layer of ginger paste at the bottom of the moxibustion implement and place the moxibustion implement on the moxibustion part.

（8）放置艾绒施灸：在姜泥上均匀铺满艾绒，自上向下点燃，待艾绒完全燃尽为1壮，继续添加艾绒点燃，如上灸取3壮，灸完3壮后取下灸具(见图2-18)。

（8）Placing moxa wool and performing moxibustion：Uniformly spread moxa wool on the ginger paste, and ignite the moxa wool from top to bottom; one zhuang is completed after the moxa wool is fully burnt out; add moxa wool and ignite again, perform moxibustion for three zhuangs in total, and remove the moxibustion implement after three zhuangs (see Fig. 2-18).

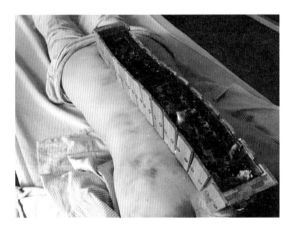

图 2-18 督灸疗法
Fig. 2-18 Du moxibustion therapy

（9）清洁灸处：将纱布连姜泥一起卷起，然后用无菌纱布轻轻擦干净灸后皮肤。

（9）Cleaning moxibustion part：Roll up the gauze together with the ginger paste, and slightly wipe up the skin by using sterile gauze.

（10）灸后处理：灸后皮肤出现红晕是正常现象，若艾火热力过强，施灸过重，皮肤易发生水疱。

（10）Post Moxibustion Treatment：After the moxibustion, the skin may show blushes, which is a normal phenomenon. If the heating power of the moxa fire is too strong, or the moxibustion is applied excessively, the skin is likely to show blisters.

小水疱无需处理，如果水疱较大以酒精棉球自上而下常规消毒3遍，用一次性无菌针头沿水疱下缘平刺,疱液自然流出,再以消毒干棉球按压干净即可。

Small blisters do not need any treatment, and big blisters may be treated: routinely sterilizing for three times from top to bottom with alcohol cotton ball, horizontally piercing along the lower edges of blisters using a disposable sterile syringe needle, waiting for blister liquid to flow out automatically, and pressing cleanly with sterilized dry cotton ball.

二、临床应用

Ⅱ. Clinical Application

（一）适用范围

（Ⅰ）Scope of Application

适用于因风寒湿邪所致的颈、肩、腰、腿等关节疼痛及软组织扭挫伤等所致的疼痛,对脊柱相关性疾病、类风湿关节炎、腰椎间盘突出症、骨性关节炎、骶髂关节炎、老年性骨质疏松症、股骨头坏死等疾病的治疗有独特效果,尤擅治疗由强直性脊柱炎所引起的疼痛,具有延缓衰老、祛除病痛、增强免疫力、平衡阴阳虚实的作用。

Du Moxibustion is applicable to joint pain of neck, shoulder, waist, leg, etc. caused by pathogenic wind, cold and dampness, and pain caused by soft tissue contusion, etc. It has unique effect on diseases related to spinal column, rheumatoid arthritis, prolapse of lumbar intervertebral disc, osteoarthritis, sacroiliitis, senile osteoporosis, femoral head necrosis, etc., and is especially good at treating pain caused by ankylosing spondylitis. It has the functions of delaying aging, removing ailments, enhancing immunity and balancing yin and yang.

（二）处方示例

（Ⅱ）Prescription Examples

1. 强直性脊柱炎　强直性脊柱炎是一种慢性、进行性、以中轴关节病变为主的炎症性关节病。

1. Ankylosing Spondylitis　Ankylosing spondylitis is a chronic, progressive and inflammatory arthropathy characterized mainly by lesions of the axial joint.

好发于青少年,病变部位主要为骶髂关节、脊柱关节、结缔组织及四肢关节。

It mostly occurs in teenagers, and sacroiliac joints, joints of vertebral column, and connective tissue and extremities joints are mostly invaded.

病理表现为椎间关节及四肢滑膜关节炎性增生纤维化、椎体纤维及韧带骨化。

The pathological manifestation includes inflammatory hyperplasia and fibrosis of intervertebral joints and extremities synovial joints, and ossification of centrum fiber and anadesma.

临床表现为脊柱弯曲畸形或直立状态,腰椎变平,颈椎前伸。

Clinical manifestation includes curvature, malformation or upright of spine, flattening of lumbar vertebra and forward protrusion of cervical vertebra.

除关节外,还可侵犯眼、肺、肾及心脏,出现相应的临床症状。

In addition to joints, ankylosing spondylitis can also invade the eye, lung, kidney and heart, with corresponding clinical symptoms.

本病属先天肾精不足,肾虚正衰,督脉空虚,复感寒湿之邪,郁而化热,而致湿热痹阻经络,迁延日久,内舍肝肾,流注关节。

This disease is caused by congenital insufficiency of kidney essence, deficiency of the kidney with weak healthy qi, and emptiness of Du meridian, and invasion into the body by pathogenic cold and dampness, with heat transformed by depression, thus causing dampness-heat blockage of meridians and collaterals and after a long period of time involving the liver and kidney, and joints.

治法:扶正祛邪、散寒止痛。

Treatment method: Strengthening healthy qi to eliminate pathogenic factors, and eliminating cold to stop pain.

操作:让患者俯卧在床上裸露背部,选取督脉大椎穴至腰俞穴,在脊柱上常规消毒,刮痧,在灸具内铺放姜泥,在姜泥上铺放一层艾绒,将灸具放置于施灸部位,点燃头、身、尾三点,让艾绒自行燃烧,燃尽后可续艾施灸,一般灸 3 壮,灸毕移去灸具,用消毒纱布轻轻擦拭皮肤。

Operation: Let the patient to lie with prone position, his/her back exposed, select the part from Dazhui point to Yaoshu point of Du meridian, perform routine sterilization on spinal column, perform scrapping, spread ginger paste in the moxibustion implement, spread a layer of moxa wool on the ginger paste, place the moxibustion implement on the moxibustion part, ignite three points, of the moxa wool head, body and tail, and let the moxa wool burn automatically. Add another layer of moxa wool to perform moxibustion after the first layer of moxa wool burns out, 3 zhuangs is used for performing moxibustion in general, remove the moxibustion implement after moxibustion is finished, and slightly wipe the skin by using sterile gauze.

2. 绝经后骨质疏松症 绝经后骨质疏松症,又称Ⅰ型骨质疏松症,属于原发性骨质疏松症,是妇女绝经后的一种常见代谢性骨病,与激素水平、遗传因素和后天因素有关,表现为骨量减少和结构破坏,致骨脆性增加,提高了骨折风险。

2. Postmenopausal Osteoporosis Postmenopausal osteoporosis, also called type Ⅰ osteoporosis, belongs to primary osteoporosis. It is a common postmenopausal metabolic bone disease for women, and is related to hormone level, genetic factors and acquired factors. Its manifestation includes osteopenia and structural deterioration which increase the bone brittleness and thus increase the risk of fracture.

该病中医称为"骨枯""骨痹""骨痿""骨极"等,疼痛是其最典型表现,可局限于腰背部,也可弥漫于周身,负重时明显加重,可以影响活动,严重时干扰翻身、行走等日常生活。

This disease is called in TCM "bone depletion", "bone Bi", "atrophic debility of bones", "bone exhaustion", etc. Its most typical manifestation is pain which may locally occur in the lumbodorsal part or generally in the body. The pain will get worse obviously when the patient bears load, and affect the movement and even interfere with the daily activities such as turning over and walking as it is serious.

治法:补益肝肾、活血止痛。

Treatment method: Tonifying the liver and kidney, and promoting blood circulation to stop pain.

操作:患者俯卧位,暴露背部,在大椎穴至腰俞穴做常规消毒,刮痧,在灸具内铺放姜泥,在姜泥上铺放一层艾绒,将灸具放置于施灸部位,点燃头、身、尾三点,让艾绒自行燃烧,燃尽后可续艾绒施灸,一般灸 3 壮,灸毕移去灸具,用消毒纱布轻轻擦拭皮肤。

Operation: Let the patient to lie in a prone position with his/her back exposed, perform routine sterilization on the part from Dazhui point to Yaoshu point, perform scrapping, spread ginger paste in the moxibustion implement, spread a layer of moxa wool on the ginger paste, place the moxibustion implement on the moxibustion part, ignite three points of the moxa wool head, body and tail, and then let the moxa wool burn automatically. Add another layer of moxa wool to perform moxibustion after the first layer of moxa wool burns out, 3 zhuangs are used for performing moxibustion in general, remove the moxibustion implement after moxibustion is finished, and slightly wipe the skin by using sterile gauze.

三、禁忌证

Ⅲ. Contraindications

1. 糖尿病、高血压、心脏病患者禁灸。

1. Du moxibustion should not be performed on patients with diabetes, hypertension and heart disease.

2. 高热患者,有出血倾向患者禁灸。

2. Du moxibustion should not be performed on patients with high fever and hemorrhagic tendency.

3. 妊娠期妇女禁灸。

3. Du moxibustion should not be performed on women during pregnancy.

4. 极度疲劳、过饥、过饱、酒醉、大汗淋漓、情绪不稳或妇女经期禁灸。

4. Moxibustion should not be performed on persons who are severely tired, too hungry, too full, drunk, drenched in sweat and unstable in emotion, or women during menstrual period.

5. 无自制能力的人,如精神病患者禁灸。

5. Du moxibustion should not be performed on persons having no self-control ability, such as psychotics.

四、注意事项

IV. Precautions

1. 治疗期间内禁食生冷辛辣、肥甘厚味、鸡、鹅、鱼腥,禁冷水洗浴、避冷风、忌房事。

1. Patients should not take raw, cold or spicy food, greasy and rich food, chicken, goose and fish. They should not take cold baths, should avoid cold wind, and should avoid sexual intercourse.

2. 体质过于虚弱者、老人、小儿及孕妇等慎用此法。

2. Persons with excessively weak constitution, the aged, children and pregnant women should be cautiously given this therapy.

五、意外情况处理方法

V. Treatment for Accidents

灸后若起水疱,则用消毒针引流,并用无菌药棉轻轻揩净,涂抹紫药水,然后覆盖一层无菌纱布,用胶布固定,直至结痂脱落为止。

If blisters appear after moxibustion, drain the liquid by using a sterilized needle, slightly wipe up by using sterile cotton, apply gentian violet, and cover a layer of sterile gauze, and fix by using adhesive tape until scab has fallen off.

参 考 文 献

References

[1] 林红,杨殿兴. 中国民间灸法绝技[M].成都:四川科学技术出版社,2007:84.

[2] 张仁,刘坚. 中国民间奇特灸法[M].上海:上海科学技术出版社,2004:74.

[3] 田丛豁,臧俊岐. 中国灸法集粹[M].沈阳:辽宁科学技术出版社,1987:71.

[4] 张奇文. 中国灸法大全[M].天津:天津科学技术出版社,1993:53.

[5] 王丽,袁卫华,蔡圣朝. 铺灸疗法的临床应用[J].针灸临床杂志,2012,28(3):35-37.

[6] 许焕芳,赵百孝. 艾灸疗法作用机理浅述[J].上海针灸杂志,2012,31(1):6-9.

[7] 王富春. 灸法捷要[M].上海:上海科学技术出版社,2009:45.

第三章 药 浴
Chapter 3 Medicated Bath

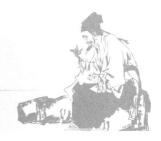

第一节 藏 药 浴
Section 1 Tibetan Medicated Bath

藏药浴是根据藏医药的基础理论而创造的一种具有藏医特色的药物外治方法。

Tibetan medicated bath is an external therapy with the characteristic of Tibetan medicine. It is created in accordance with the basic theories of traditional Tibetan medical science.

由于它治疗适应证广,安全无痛苦,疗效好,深受广大藏族人民欢迎。

It has received warm welcome from the Tibetan people due to its wide range of treatment indication, safety, painlessness and good efficacy.

藏族人民自古以来居住在高原地区,在长期的生产生活实践中,很早就认识到沐浴有利于身体健康。

Tibetan people have lived in highlands since ancient times, and during long-term working and life practices, they have realized very early that bathing is beneficial to people's health.

在此基础上,藏医根据"三因学说"和"五元学说"理论,从理、法、方、药上不断更新、完善,结合藏族地区独特的地理环境、气候条件和发病规律,从而创造了藏医独特的"药汁浸泡型"外治方法,并逐步总结出一套完备、系统的药浴理论和技术。

On this basis, the Tibetan medicine has been constantly updated and perfected from aspects of the theory, therapy, recipe and medicine according to the "Theory of Three Types of Disease Causes" and "Theory of Five Types of Disease

Causes". On the basis of the unique geographical environment, weather condition and incidence rules of diseases in the Tibetan region, the Tibetan unique external therapy of "Medicine Liquid Immersion Type" was created, and a set of complete and systematic theories and techniques is gradually summarized.

一、藏药浴的作用机制

Ⅰ. Action Mechanism of Tibetan Medicated Bath

藏药浴中药物的有效成分通过毛囊壁 - 汗腺 - 皮脂腺 - 角质层细胞而被毛细血管网吸收。

Active ingredients of the medicine are absorbed by the capillary network via hair follicle wall-sweat gland-sebaceous gland-horny layer cell.

药液的有效成分通过上述通道进入人体的组织器官发挥独特的作用,可以调节改善组织功能。

These active ingredients enter tissues and organs of the human body via the above channel to play a unique role to regulate and improve the tissue function.

药液的水温能使体内外温度升高,伴随毛孔开放的同时,增强各组织器官的活动与循环能力,使滞留于体内的病毒、病菌通过毛孔排出体外,达到净化血液、软化瘀结、清除组织滑膜水肿、恢复关节功能的治疗作用。

The temperature of medicinal liquid can rise both in-vivo and in-vitro temperatures, open pores on body surface, and improve the activity and circulation capabilities of tissues and organs, so as to expel viruses and bacteria retained in the body through the pores and achieve the therapeutic effects of purifying blood, softening blood stasis, eliminating tissue synovial membrane edema and recovering joint function.

现代科研证明,藏药浴能促进血液循环,加强机体代谢,提高白细胞吞噬能力,还能调节神经功能,增强免疫力。

Modern scientific research demonstrates that the Tibetan medicated bath can promote blood circulation, strengthen body metabolism, enhance the phagocytosis of white blood cells, regulate neurological function and boost immunity.

二、藏药浴的组成

Ⅱ. Composition of Tibetan Medicated Bath

"五味甘露"是藏药浴的基础配方。

"Five-taste sweet dew" is the basis formula of Tibetan medicated bath.

包括藏麻黄(丁香)、水柏枝(诃子)、圆柏(旃檀)、黄花杜鹃(杜鹃花)和灰蒿(水生)五种药物。

"Five-taste sweet dew" includes five drugs: ephedra saxatilis (clove), german tamarisk (medicine terminalia fruit), sabina chinensis (sandalwood), rhododendron lutescens (rhododendron) and grey wormwood herb (hydrophyte).

现代藏医在此基础上,根据不同的疾病,辨证加以藏红花、三七、天麻、灵芝、冬虫夏草等多种药材,达到更好的防病治病目的。

On this basis, multiple medicinal materials such as saffron, pseudo-ginseng, tall gastrodia tuber, glossy ganoderma and Chinese caterpillar fungus are added according to syndrome differentiation of different diseases, achieving better effect for prevention and care of disease.

三、藏药浴功效

Ⅲ. Efficacy of Tibetan Medicated Bath

(一) 保健作用
(Ⅰ) Health Care

藏药浴疗法可以通过皮肤吸收药物从而改善皮肤生态系统,增强新陈代谢,改善血液运行状态。

The Tibetan medicated bath therapy, through skin absorption, can improve the ecological system of the skin, enhance metabolism and improve blood flow.

在温热环境下,皮下血管会扩张充血,心率加快,新陈代谢旺盛,对心血管的功能有促进作用,也是一种被动性的养生过程,以达到保健目的。

In a warm environment, subcutaneous blood vessels will expand and congest, the heart rate will increase, the metabolism will become strong, thus reinforcing cardiovascular function. The Tibetan medicated bath is also a passive life cultivation process, so as to achieve the purpose of health care.

（二）调理内分泌

（Ⅱ）Endocrine Regulation

藏药浴所用的天然草药,通过炮制发酵加温,在热能的作用下,透过人体的皮肤孔窍进入机体,通过穴位经络发挥作用。

The natural herbal medicine, after being processed, fermented and heated, can enter the human body through the orifices under the action of thermal energy and play its therapeutic effect through the acupoints, meridians and collaterals.

经多年的临床研究证明,藏医的医学观点,"因人而异,辨证配伍",由藏医医生通过传统的诊断方法,针对性地开具浴疗配方,平衡人体体液的酸碱度,有效改善内分泌失调的症状。

Clinical research of many years has verified that the Tibetan medicine has been sticking to the medical view of "varying from person to person, and compatibility based on syndrome differentiated". Tibetan doctors give a targeted prescription for therapeutic bath based on a traditional diagnosis, aiming to balance the acid-alkali level of human body fluids and effectively relieve the endocrine dyscrasia.

同时其头部的局部药浴,因其配方中有很多药具有活血成分,并含有多种微量元素,对改善发质、生发、养发起到直接作用。

Meanwhile, the local medicated bath for the head is capable of improving hair quality, growing hair and nourishing hair due to the blood circulation promoting ingredients and various trace elements contained in the medicine.

（三）排除身体毒素和提高免疫力

（Ⅲ）Removal of Toxins and Improvement of Immunity

藏医认为,饮食搭配、环境、药物用法不当或过度使用等均会造成毒素的沉积。毒素不能及时更新代谢,成为隐藏于身体中最危险的物质。

The Tibetan medicine considers that factors of diet, environment, and improper or excessive drug use may result in toxin deposition. These toxins cannot be metabolized in time, and then they will be the most dangerous substances in the body.

藏医有种说法叫"人所患疾,皆为吃而生,马病皆因累而生",所以这就是人体需要排毒的原因所在。

There is a saying in Tibetan medicine:All diseases of a person are due to diet,and all diseases of a horse are due to exhaustion. This is why the human body needs to remove toxins.

藏药浴的排毒作用,已被藏医近千年的临床实践所证明。

The function of expelling toxins of the Tibetan medicated bath has been proved by nearly one thousand years of clinical practices of the Tibetan medicine.

藏药浴中的药物,很多具有活血化瘀、滋润肌肤、除风祛湿、解除毒素的功效成分,可以有效分解血管中的沉积物质,改善血管壁的自然功能及弹性度。

The medicine used for Tibetan medicated bath contains a number of active ingredients capable of promoting blood circulation,removing blood stasis, moisturizing the skin,dispelling wind and eliminating dampness,and expelling toxins,so it may effectively decompose substances deposited in the blood vessels and improve the natural function and degree of elasticity of the vessel wall.

同时,在藏药浴的热能作用与药物的发汗作用下,这些分解后的有害物质,如多余的胆固醇、多余的脂肪、尿酸和瘀血等人体毒素,可以随着汗液与其他体液排出体外。同时藏药浴还可以促进胃肠道的蠕动,排出宿便。

Meanwhile,under the thermal action of the Tibetan medicated bath and inducing perspiration of the medicine,hazardous substances such as redundant cholesterol,redundant fat,uric acid and blood stasis can be excreted to the outside of the body along with the sweat and other body fluids. In addition,the Tibetan medicated bath can promote the peristalsis of gastrointestinal tract to eliminate the stool.

藏药浴的药物透过皮下孔窍进入毛细血管,再通过血液周身循环,进入人体的各个组织、器官,通过热能下的体液置换作用,达到"吐故纳新、排除毒素"的核心作用。

The medicine enters the capillary vessels via subcutaneous orifices,circulates all over the human body along with blood,enters various tissues and organs and plays the role of getting rid of the stale and taking in the fresh and expelling the toxins through the body fluid displacement in the thermal environment.

（四）改善疲劳，提高精神状态
（Ⅳ）Fatigue Relief and Improvement of Mental State

藏药浴能减轻或解除疲劳、调节神经衰弱等症状，尤其对高度精神压力、精神紧张、长期失眠的脑力工作者是一种集调理、放松、解疲、保健为一体的疗效显著的治疗方式。

The Tibetan medicated bath can alleviate or relieve fatigue and modulate the neurasthenia. It integrates the conditioning, relaxing, fatigue relief and health care, and is an effective therapy for brain workers suffering from high mental stress, psychentonia and chronic insomnia.

在藏医理论中，被归纳出的"三因不和""毒素沉积"的现象，通常表现为体内沉积的、对身体有害的废物过多，血液氧分不足（气血不足），而影响部分脏器功能，这与现代医学中的"亚健康理论"不谋而合。

In the theory of Tibetan medicine, the phenomena of "Discomfort due to Three Types of Disease Causes" and "Toxin Deposition" often manifest as too much insalubrious waste deposited in the human body, and insufficient blood oxygen (insufficiency of qi and blood), which affect partial functions of visceral organs. These phenomena coincide with the sub-health theory of the modern medicine.

通过近几十年的临床观察，藏药浴对人体精神状态有明显改善作用，它的原理在于通过药浴，松弛紧张疲劳的全身神经，以逸治劳，使全身神经、肌肉充分放松，达到身体各系统相互平衡的目的。

As has been observed for several tens of years, the Tibetan medicated bath can dramatically improve the mental state of a person. It works because the medicated bath may relax the frayed and tired nerves and muscles of the whole body, so as to balance various body systems.

（五）提高睡眠质量
（Ⅴ）Improvement of Sleep Quality

藏药浴对睡眠的改善和加深有特殊作用，藏药具有安神、活血、通络、解疲的作用。

The Tibetan medicated bath is capable of improving and deepening sleep because the Tibetan medicine has the functions of relieving uneasiness of the mind, promoting blood circulation, dredging meridians and alleviating physical fatigue.

藏药浴通过渗透作用,使全身的毛细血管同时受到药物浸润热能和药效双重的作用,使得机体及神经高度放松,继而使纷乱的大脑思绪平静,通常一个疗程药浴结束后,受浴患者一般都可以获得高质量的睡眠。

Through the medicine penetration, capillary vessels of the whole body can get the dual actions of the thermal energy and the pharmaceutical effect. The Tibetan medicated bath can highly relax the body and the nerves and calm down emotions. Generally after a course of treatment, the patient can get a sleep of high-quality.

四、藏药浴的适应证

Ⅳ. Indications of Tibetan Medicated Bath

《四部医典·后续部》中记载:"四肢强直或挛急、跛跷、疖痈、炭疽、新旧疮疡炎肿、各种皮肤病、妇女产后风、弓腰驼背关节变形、肌肤之间黄水充斥及各种隆病等均属藏药浴的治疗范围。"随着临床对藏药浴技术的广泛应用和科研的不断深入,藏药浴的治疗范围已拓展到藏医各个临床领域。

The *Subsequent Parts of the Four Medical Canons* records that "Orthocolosis or hypertonicity of the limbs, cyllopodia, furuncle and carbuncle, anthrax, old and new swellings and ulcers, various skin diseases, puerperal fever, humpback and arthrentasis, yellow pus between skin and muscle and various blood diseases are all within the scope of treatment of the Tibetan medicated bath." With the extensive use of the Tibetan medicated bath and the constant deepening of scientific research, the scope of treatment of the Tibetan medicated bath has been expanded to various clinical areas of the Tibetan medicine.

1. 风湿免疫系统疾病,如风湿、类风湿关节炎、痛风、强直性脊柱炎、产后风等。

1. Rheumatic immune systemic diseases, such as rheumatism, rheumatoid arthritis, gout, ankylosing spondylitis and puerperal fever.

2. 骨科、神经科疾病,如骨质增生、骨性关节炎、颈椎病、腰椎间盘突出、肩周炎、各种软组织损伤、骨质疏松、骨折恢复期、头痛、头晕、脑梗死后遗症等。

2. Orthopedic and neurological diseases, such as hyperosteogeny, osteoarthritis, cervical spondylosis, lumbar interverte-bral disc herniation, scapulohumeral periarthritis, various soft tissue injuries, osteoporosis, fracture recovery period, headache, dizziness and cerebral infarction sequel.

3. 皮肤科疾病,如银屑病、局限性硬皮病、过敏性皮炎、日光性皮炎、神经性皮炎、鱼鳞病、荨麻疹、湿疹等。

3. Dermatological diseases, such as psoriasis, scleroderma circumscriptum, allergic dermatitis, solar dermatitis, neurodermatitis, ichthyosis, urticaria, eczema, etc.

随着对藏药浴的深入挖掘和不断研究,藏药浴的治疗范围已拓展到治疗妇科疾病和保健美容等更多领域,并取得了良好的效果。

With deep digging and continuous research on Tibetan medicated bath, its scope of treatment has been expended to more fields with satisfying results, such as gynecological diseases, health care, and beauty.

五、藏药浴的禁忌证及注意事项

Ⅴ. Precautions and Contraindications of Tibetan Medicated Bath

1. 严重的心脏病、高血压、传染病、水肿、妊娠及妇女行经期禁浴。

1. Patients with severe heart diseases, hypertension, infectious diseases and edema, and women during pregnancy and menstrual period should not be allowed to take the bath.

2. 女性患者月经结束 3~4 天后开始治疗。

2. Women may take the bath 3-4 days after the menstruation.

3. 患者治疗 1 疗程后间隔 15~30 天可进行第 2 疗程。

3. After the first course of treatment, patients may take the second course of treatment after an interval of 15-30 days.

4. 治疗期间要加强保暖,避风寒,注意休息,适度锻炼,加强营养,忌食刺激性、寒凉食物。

4. Patients should pay more attention to keep warm, avoid cold, take good

rest, exercise moderately, eat nutritious food and avoid eating spicy and cold food during the treatment.

六、藏药浴后的护理

Ⅵ. Nursing after Tibetan Medicated Bath

进行藏药浴后,患者应平躺于暖房,用被子盖好全身及手足,最好用毛巾或帽子遮盖头部。

After taking the Tibetan medicated bath, the patients should lie flat in a warm house and cover the whole body and hands and feet with a quilt. It is best to cover the head of the patients with a towel or hat.

由于药浴期间会出汗导致大量水分丢失,身体消耗量大,患者有时会出现恶心、头晕等症状。

Patients will perspire during medicated bath and thus lose much water and consume much energy, so they sometime may have such symptoms as nausea and dizziness.

如出现上述症状时患者应缓慢出浴,休息片刻后适当饮用淡盐水,叮嘱患者多吃新鲜蔬菜及高蛋白、高营养、高热量易消化的食物,禁食生、冷、辛辣食物。

When the above symptoms appear, the patients should come out from the bath slowly and after a short break, drink light salt water. Also the patients should be instructed to eat more fresh vegetables and digestible food with high protein, high nutrition and high calorie and should not eat raw, cold and spicy food.

出院时应向家属交代患者需要在家休息 2~3 周,鼓励病人积极进行体能锻炼,全身保暖,避免受凉,要适当运动,不宜过度劳累,休息期内不宜洗澡,注意保暖,防止着凉引起不良反应,避免潮湿。

When patients leave the hospital, it should be made clear to their relatives that the patients should stay at home for 2-3 weeks and they are encouraged to take physical exercises actively, and keep the whole body warm, exercise moderately, avoid overstrain, avoid bathing, keep warm during rest period, avoid cold to avoid adverse reaction, and avoid dampness.

参 考 文 献
References

［1］段利学.藏药浴与养生保健［J］.中国民族医药杂志,2014,20(6):71-73.
［2］金学英.藏医特色药浴疗法综论［J］.亚太传统医药,2010,6(3):101-102.

第二节 瑶 药 浴
Section 2 Yao Medicated Bath

瑶药浴是瑶族民间用以抵御风寒、消除疲劳、防治疾病的传统行为。

The Yao medicated bath is a traditional method used by the Yao people to withstand cold, relieve fatigue and prevent and cure diseases.

瑶药浴以多种植物药为配方,经过烧煮制成药水,放入杉木桶,人坐桶内熏浴浸泡,让药液渗透五脏六腑、全身经络,达到祛风除湿、活血化瘀、排汗排毒的功效。

Yao people collect various plants and put them into cedar barrel after decocting them into medicine liquid. A patient sits inside the barrel to let the medicine liquid penetrate into the internal organs and whole body meridians and collaterals to realize the efficacy of dispelling wind and eliminating dampness, promoting blood circulation and removing blood stasis, and perspiring sweat and excreting toxins.

瑶族医药作为瑶族历史传统文化的一个重要组成部分,有其鲜明的民族特色及用药特点。

Yao medicine, as an important part of Yao historical traditional culture, has distinctive national features and medication characteristics.

其药浴疗法,已成为瑶族人民健身、治病、益寿延年的习俗。

Its medicated bath therapy has become the customs of keeping fitness, curing diseases and promoting longevity of Yao people.

自古以来,瑶族人民多喜依高山而居,外出或劳作归家后,必先用热水或热药液洗浴,如有客自远方来,首先招待客人的就是热水泡澡。

From ancient times to the present, Yao people always prefer to live on or around the mountains. After returning home from going out or working, Yao people would certainly take a bath with hot water or hot medicinal liquid. When there is a visitor coming, Yao people will entertain the visitor with a hot bath.

其原因是山区日照时数少,日夜温差较大,相对湿度较大,出门难免跋山涉水,极易感受风寒湿邪,病后就医不便,多采用药浴法预防或治疗。

The reason is that there are short duration of sunshine, large temperature difference between day and night, and high relative humidity in the mountain area. People living there always climb mountains and cross rivers, and are easy to get sick due to wind-cold-dampness evil. It is inconvenient for the patient to seek medical advice, Yao people take medicated bath to prevent or cure diseases.

此法代代相传,已成为当地人民的生活习惯,也形成了一系列具有瑶族特色的防病、治病方药。

This method is handed down from generation to generation, and has become a living habit of the local people. In addition, a series of prescriptions for disease prevention and curing with characteristics of Yao nationality have been formed.

庞桶药浴是瑶药浴最大的特点。

A huge barrel is the biggest characteristic of Yao medicated bath.

人们采集新鲜的草药,用水煎煮后,倒入一个庞大的木桶中进行洗浴,由于运用的桶比较庞大,故称为庞桶药浴。

Yao people collect fresh herbal medicine, decoct it in water, and pour the medicine liquid in a huge barrel. Because the barrel used for bathing is relatively large, the Yao medicated bath is also called the huge-barrel medicated bath.

庞桶药浴在疾病的防治中具有简、便、廉、验的优势。

The huge-barrel medicated bath has the advantages of simpleness, convenience, low price and effectiveness in terms of prevention and curing of diseases.

另外,庞桶药浴安全,对皮肤无过敏、毒性反应等不良作用。

In addition, the huge-barrel medicated bath is safe and does not result in cutaneous allergy or cutaneous toxicity.

一、瑶药浴的作用机制

I. Action Mechanism of Yao Medicated Bath

瑶药浴作为外治法的一种,与内治法的作用机制殊途同归。

As an external therapy, the Yao medicated bath has the same action mechanism as that of the internal therapy.

从中医学的角度来说,《素问·阴阳应象大论》云:"其有邪者,渍形以为汗。"在我国古代就认为可以用汤液浸渍取汗,以达到祛邪的目的。

From the perspective of TCM, it is recorded in *Plain Questions-Theory of Yin and Yang* that "for patients falling ill due to the pathogenic factor, immersing the body with hot water to make them sweaty". In ancient China, it was believed that immersing the body with hot water to induce perspiration can achieve the purpose of eliminating pathogens.

人体的五脏六腑、四肢百骸、腠理毛窍,无不相通。

The internal organs, limbs and bones, and striae and orifices of the human body are all communicated with each other.

通过药浴可以使药物进入腠理,以达病所,从而起到"祛风除湿、舒筋活血、解毒通络、强身健体"的作用。

By a medicated bath, medicine enters the striae and reaches the diseased part to achieve the purposes of dispelling wind and eliminating dampness, relieving rigidity of muscles and promoting blood circulation, dispelling toxins and dredging collaterals, and strengthening the body.

另外,瑶药浴还可以调节人体免疫功能,增强机体抗病能力。

Moreover, the Yao medicated bath is capable of regulating the immune function of human body and enhancing the body resistance against diseases.

从现代医学的角度来看,皮肤面积大,具有吸收、渗透、分泌、排泄等多种功能,在人体的生理病理方面发挥着重要的作用。

From the perspective of modern medicine, a person has a large area of skin which has the functions of absorption, penetration, secretion, excretion and the like,playing an important function in physiology and pathology.

皮肤内的神经末梢及特殊感受器,可以调节神经、体液、循环功能,改善相应组织器官的活动以增强机体的抗病和修复能力。

Nerve endings and special receptors in the skin regulate the nerves,body fluids and circulatory function and improve the activities of the corresponding tissues and organs to enhance the disease resistance and recovery capability of the body.

此外,皮肤的分泌、排泄、代谢功能参与机体对尿酸、尿素、一些无机盐类及体内毒素等代谢废物的排泄,即瑶医所谓"解毒排毒",瑶药浴正是利用了皮肤这些功能来防治疾病。

In addition,the functions of secretion,excretion and metabolism of the skin participate in the excretion of metabolic wastes such as uric acid,urea,some inorganic salts and toxins in the body. That is so-called "detoxification" of Yao medicine. Yao medicated bath does utilize these functions of the skin to prevent and cure diseases.

二、瑶药浴的起源

Ⅱ. Origin of Yao Medicated Bath

瑶族一直以来都是一个迁徙的民族,瑶族人民一般居住在湿度极大常年云雾缭绕的高坡上,相传瑶族祖先在迁徙过程中,极易引发风湿、伤寒等疾病。

Yao people have always been a migrating ethnic group and they generally live in the high slopes with high humidity and perennial mists. Tradition has it that Yao's ancestors were very easily to get such diseases as rheumatism and typhoid.

因缺医少药,长期以来,生活在深山密林中的瑶族同胞,对原始森林中的野生藤木感知最为深刻。

Due to shortage of doctors and medicine,Yao compatriots who live in deep mountains and forests for a long time have deep perception on the wild rattans in primeval forests.

他们为了生存,利用大自然赋予的各种植被进行治病防病和保健养生,抵御病毒侵害,形成了防病、保健、养生的生活理念。

For their survival, Yao compatriots use vegetation given by the nature to prevent and cure diseases, preserve health and resist invasions by bacteria and viruses. They have formed a life concept of disease prevention, health care and life cultivation.

在漫长的岁月和长期的劳动中,他们经常采大山之灵草、深山之鲜药加水熬煮,用木桶浸泡洗浴。

During the long years and long-term laboring, Yao compatriots collected herbal medicines from remote mountains, decocted them in water and held the medicine liquid in a barrel for soaking bath.

因瑶族缺少文字的记载,因此瑶族药浴具体起源时间无法考证。最早的记载瑶族善用医的文献可追溯到宋代,宋人周去非的《岭外代答》卷七说:"零陵香,出瑶洞及静江、融州、象州。凡深山木阴沮洳之地,皆可种也。"这说明,当时瑶族的医药文化知识已经相当丰富。

Due to lack of literature records, the exact origin time of Yao medicated bath cannot be verified. The earliest references which record that Yao people are good at medical treatment can be traced back to Song Dynasty. Volume Ⅶ of *Ling Wai Dai Da* by Zhou Qufei at the Song Dynasty said: "The holy basil comes from Yaodong, Jingjiang, Rongzhou and Xiangzhou. Wherever there are remote mountains and wood-land shadow in the wet land, the holy basil can be planted." This explains that Yao's medical culture knowledge at that time was rather abundant.

三、瑶药浴的药物组成

Ⅲ. Composition of Yao Medicated Bath

瑶药浴的常用草药有上百种,而且根据不同时节和不同地域、不同习惯所选择的药物也不同。

There are hundreds of kinds of herbal medicines frequently used for Yao medicated bath, and depending on the season, the region and the custom, different medicines can be selected.

常用于防治风湿病的药物有入山虎、上山虎、下山虎、爬山虎、黑老虎、猛老虎、毛老虎、走马风、九层风、龙骨风、过山风、九节风、牛耳风、四方风、大散骨风、小散骨风、血风、麻骨风、小节风、五层风、白风、破骨风、五爪风、大钻、九龙钻、小红钻、穿山钻、黄钻、梅花钻、双钩钻、穿破石、牛膝、白纸扇、一块瓦、白藤、杜仲、珠芽艾麻、血党、白藤、五指通、枫荷桂、红接骨草、铺地蜈蚣、五加皮、防风、伸筋草、一包针、半枫荷、四方钻、紫九牛、毛冬青、铜钻等。

Medicines frequently used to prevent and cure the rheumatism include: cuatgv gemh ndomh maauh, faaux gemh ndomh maauh, njiec gemh ndomh maauh, Japanese creeper stem, radix kadsurae coccineae, mongv ndomh maauh, bei ndomh maauh, yiangh maz buerng, nduoh nzangh buerng, luerngh mbungv buerng, guiex gemh buerng, glabrous sarcandra herb, nqu ngh meih nomh buerng, cissus pteroclada hayata, domh nzaamxm bungv buerng, fiuv nzaanx mbungv buerng, nziaamh buerng, mah mbungv buerng, xiaojiefeng, ba nzangh buerng, baifeng, paaix mbungv buerng, ba nqiuv buerng, donh nzunx, juov luerngh nzunx, finv hongh nzunx, chuanshanzuan, wiangh nzunx, meihuazuan, sungh diux nzunx, cudrania cochinchinensis, twotoothed achyranthes root, Buddha's lamp twig and leaf, asarum insigne, all-grass of Fourfinger Rattanpalm, eucommia bark, laportea bulbifera, ardisia brevicaulis, all-grass of Fourfinger Rattanpalm, cortex schefflerae octophyllae, root of common sassafras, didymocarpus hedyotideus Chun, lycopodium cernuum, acanthopanax, divaricate saposhnikovia root, common clubmoss herb, compositae bidens pilosa, pterospermum heterophyllum hance, feix bung nzunx, maerng juon nqungh, pubescent holly root, nongh nzunx, etc.

常用于防治妇科疾病的药物有益母草、大枫药、过江龙、走马胎、大血藤、海风藤、鸡血藤、钩藤、桂枝、透骨消、野艾、络石藤等。

Medicines frequently used to prevent and cure gynecological diseases include: motherwort herb, Dafengyao, stem of climbing entada, giantleaf ardisia rhizome, sargentgloryvine stem, piper kadsura, suberect spatholobus stem, grambir plant nod, cassia twig, ground ivy, wild wormwood, Chinese starjasmine stem, etc.

常用于防治外感疾病的药物有六月雪、旱田草、青蒿全草、野菊花、忍冬藤、山芝麻、桉树叶、马鞭草、牛筋草、鸡眼草、木防己叶、酢浆草、桃树叶、鸡矢藤、醉鱼草等。

Medicines frequently used to prevent and cure exogenous diseases include: snow of june herb, dry falsepimpernel herb, sweet wormwood herb, wild chrysanthemum flower, honeysuckle stem, screwtree root, eucalyptus leaf, vervain, eleusine indica, common lespedeza, southern fangchi root leaf, creeping oxalis, peach leaf, Chinese fevervine herb and root, buddleia, etc.

常用于防治皮肤病的药物有艾叶、葫芦卷须、柚子树叶、黄皮果枝叶、苦楝树皮、西河柳、荆芥、桃子树叶、香菜、雄鸡毛、鲜韭菜、浮萍、九里明、蒲公英、桑叶、夏枯草、稻草灰等。

Medicines frequently used to prevent and cure skin diseases include: argy wormwood leaves, calabash tendril, grapefruit leaf, branch and leaf of Chinese wampee fruit, chinaberry bark, Chinese tamarisk twig, fineleaf schizonepeta herb, peach leaf, coriander, chicken feather, fresh chives, common ducksmeat herb, senecio scandens, dandelion, folium mori, common selfheal fruit-spike, rice-straw ash, etc.

四、瑶药浴的功效

Ⅳ. Efficacy of Yao Medicated Bath

瑶药浴是在瑶医盈亏平衡理论的指导下进行的。

Yao medicated bath is conducted under the guidance of excess-deficiency balance theory of Yao medicine.

盈亏平衡理论作为瑶医的核心病机，很好地指导着瑶医防治疾病。

As the core pathogenesis of Yao medicine, the theory of excess-deficiency balance directs the Yao doctors to prevent and cure diseases.

瑶医认为在瑶药浴前，首先要判断机体的盈亏平衡状态，盈则满，满则溢，溢则病。

Yao medicine considers that the excess-deficiency balance of human body should be firstly determined before the medicated bath. Excess causes fullness, fullness causes overflow, and overflow causes illness.

亏则虚，虚则损，损则病。

In a similar way, deficiency causes insufficiency, insufficiency causes harm, and harm causes illness.

其次，在瑶药浴的运用上要遵循"风亏打盈"的原则，做到"盈则消之，亏则补之",以打药为主来治疗盈证,以风药为主治疗亏证。

Second, the use of Yao medicated bath should follow the principle of "dispelling the excess and replenishing the insufficiency", which mainly uses the "laxative medicines" to cure excess diseases and uses the "wind medicines" to cure insufficiency diseases.

在具体药物的运用方面,要根据脏腑盈亏的不同,分别选择不同的打药和风药,或者根据需要以打药和风药相配伍来达到防治疾病的目的。

Depending on the excess or insufficiency state of zang-fu organs of the body, different kinds of laxative or wind medicines can be selected or combined to prevent and cure the diseases.

如治疗盈证多以打药"五虎"为主,对于亏证则以风药"九牛"为主,而对于瘀血内阻、风湿阻痹等疾病则以通达经脉、透利关节的"十八钻"为主。

For example, to cure excess diseases, five kinds of laxative medicines with "maauh" in their name are mainly selected; to cure insufficiency diseases, nine kinds of wind medicines with "ngongh" in their name are mainly selected; to cure internal stagnation of the blood and rheumatism, eighteen kinds of medicines with "nzunx" in their name are selected to dredge the meridians and joints.

(一) 治疗作用
(I) Therapeutic Effect

瑶药浴主要具有以下几种治疗功效:一是具有舒筋活络、祛风止痛之功效,常用上山虎、下山虎、走马风、九层风、龙骨风、桑寄生、豨莶草、独活、牛膝、干杜仲、宽筋藤、当归、姜黄、续断、两面针、麻黄、鸡血藤等,适用于风湿周身骨痛、腰膝酸软。

The Yao medicated bath mainly has the following therapeutic effects: Firstly, medicines with the effects of relieving rigidity of muscles, activating collaterals, expelling pathogenic wind and relieving pains such as faaux gemh ndomh maauh, njiec gemh ndomh maauh, yiangh maz buerng, nduoh nzangh buerng, luerngh mbungv buerng, parasite scurrula, herba siegesbeckiae, doubleteeth pubescent angelica root, twotoothed achyranthes root, dry eucommia ulmoides, caulis tinosporae sinensis, Chinese angelica, turmeric, teasel root, shinyleaf pricklyash root,Chinese ephedra and suberect spatholobus stem are used to cure rheumatism, bone pain,and soreness and weakness of waist and knees.

二是具有降压之功效,常用豨莶草、罗布麻叶、夜交藤、牡蛎、吴茱萸等,适用于高血压。

Secondly,medicines with the effects of lowering blood pressure such as herba siegesbeckiae,dogbane leaf,tuber fleeceflower stem,oyster shell and medicinal evodia fruit are used to cure the hypertension.

三是扶正祛邪、益气固表之功效,常用鲜薄荷、荆芥、六月雪、旱田草、青蒿全草、鱼腥草等,适用于日常流行性感冒发热。

Thirdly,medicines with the effects of strengthening the body resistance and eliminating pathogenic factors,and invigorating qi for consolidating superficies such as fresh mint,fineleaf schizonepeta herb,snow of june herb,dry falsepimpernel herb,sweet wormwood herb and heartleaf houttuynia herb are used to cure epidemic influenza and fever.

四是活血化瘀的功效,常用苏木、松节、赤芍、红花、没药等,治疗外伤瘀血、跌打肿痛。

Fourthly,medicines with the effects of promoting blood circulation and removing blood stasis such as sappan wood,pine nodular branch,peony root, safflower and myrrh are used to cure traumatic stasis and pain and swelling from injuries.

五是祛湿止痒、收涩敛疮、化腐生肌,常用柚子树叶、苦楝树皮、西河柳、荆芥、桃子树叶、雄鸡毛、浮萍、九里明、稻草灰等,治疗各类皮肤病。

Fifthly,medicines with the effects of removing dampness to relieve itching, inducing astringency and promoting wound healing,and removing slough and promoting regeneration of the tissue such as grapefruit leaf,chinaberry bark, Chinese tamarisk twig,fineleaf schizonepeta herb,peach leaf,chicken feather, common ducksmeat herb,senecio scandens and rice-straw ash are used to cure skin diseases of all sorts.

（二）养生保健作用
（Ⅱ）Life Cultivation and Health Care Effect
瑶药浴所用药物因地制宜,功能多种多样,有清热解毒、祛风散寒、舒筋活络、滋补气血等。

According to local conditions, medicines with the functions of clearing away heat and resolving toxins material, expelling wind and removing cold, relieving rigidity of muscles and activating collaterals, and nourishing blood and invigorating qi are selected for the medicated bath.

药浴时,常根据不同对象、不同季节或不同疾病选择不同药物。

According to difference in recipient, season or disease, different medicines are selected.

通常新生儿及产后妇女多选用温补的药物,比如大血藤、五指毛桃、九节风、鸭仔风、穿破石、杜仲藤等,这样可预防产妇及新生儿的各种感染,滋补气血,促进产妇子宫复旧。

Generally, warming and invigorating medicines such as sargentgloryvine stem, hairy fig, glabrous sarcandra herb, apc dorn buerng, cudrania cochinchinensis and root or stem of smallflower parabarium are selected for newborn babies and postpartum women to prevent the infection, nourish blood and invigorate qi, and promote uterine recovery.

产后药浴,人们称之为"月里药浴",许多瑶族妇女,产后经过药浴等调养保健,产后 10 天左右就能上山参加体力劳动,同时新生儿往往有随母药浴的习惯。

Postnatal medicated bath is also called the lying-in medicated bath. With the help of medicated bath and other recovery and health care methods, many women of Yao nationality can take part in physical labor about ten days after parturition, and often take the medicated bath together with their babies.

劳动后淋雨受寒,也要进行药浴,可起到温中散寒、舒筋活络及恢复体力、预防风湿的作用。

After being exposed to the rain and affected by cold, Yao people also take a medicated bath to warm the spleen and stomach to dispel cold, relieve rigidity of muscles, activate collaterals, relieve fatigue, and prevent rheumatism.

常选药物为老姜、米酒、大发散、小发散、桃树叶、青蒿等。

Medicines commonly used include old ginger, rice wine, Parish's Ironweed, xiaofasan,peach leaf,sweet wormwood herb,etc.

老年人也很注重药浴,一般多用活血温补之药,如大钻、小钻、大血藤、扶芳藤、青春藤等。

The elderly of Yao nationality also appreciate the medicated bath,and they usually use the warming and invigorating medicines to promote blood circulation, such as donh nzunx,fiuv nzunx,sargentgloryvine stem,euonymus fortune and Chinese ivy stem.

五、瑶药浴的操作方法

Ⅴ. Operation Method of Yao Medicated Bath

在瑶族人家到处可见到用杉木做成的高 1m、宽 0.6m、长 0.7m 的大木桶,这便是用药水洗澡的"庞桶",又称为"黄桶"。

Big barrels(1m in height,0.6m in width and 0.7m in length)made of cedarwood are seen everywhere in Yao's families,and they are the so-called "huge barrel"(also referred to as "yellow barrel")used for bathing with medicinal liquid.

庞桶浴将采集到的新鲜草药,捆成小捆,1∶7 放入大锅中煎煮至沸腾约 30 分钟,将沸水倒入木桶中,然后兑入冷水,使水温保持在 40℃左右,进行洗浴,水温降低后要及时补充热水,避免受寒。

In "huge barrel bath",the collected fresh herbs are bunched into wisps and put into the boiler to be boiled for about 30 minutes with a 1∶7 ratio,and then people take the bath after some cold water is added to keep the water temperature at about 40℃. In case of catching cold,hot water should be added timely when water temperature drops.

每次洗浴时间约 30 分钟,10 天为 1 个疗程。

One bathing time lasts for about 30 minutes and one course of treatment contains 10 days.

根据瑶族地区的风俗,多为全家洗浴,先客后主,老幼妇孺优先。

According to the local custom of Yao's region,the whole family take the bath together in most cases,usually hosts take after guests and the old,children and women take precedence.

六、瑶药浴的注意事项及禁忌

Ⅵ. Precautions and Contraindication of Yao Medicated Bath

1. 浸泡药浴前、中、后应适当补充水分,也可以喝淡盐水、糖水。

1. Before, during and after the medicated bath, people should moderately drink light salt water and sweet water.

2. 浸泡场地注意室内温度,通风良好,不可蓄意吹风,以免受寒。

2. The bathing area should be well controlled on temperature and well ventilated, but no deliberate expose of blowing wind in case of catching cold.

3. 起浴后皮肤表面发红,并持续 30 分钟至 2 小时的发汗,均属正常的药效作用。

3. People's skin surface will turn red after the bath and they will sweat for 30 minutes to 2 hours, which are all normal medicine efficacies.

4. 有中度高低血压病史、心脏功能稍差者应在家人陪伴下进行,注意场地通风,每次浸泡时间不宜太长(3~6 分钟),如浸泡过程中感到心动过速或呼吸急促时,应缓慢起身于通风良好处稍作休息,等恢复后再次浸泡,一般分 2~3 次浸泡即可。

4. Those who have a history of moderate hypertension or hypotension and have poor cardiac function should take the bath in the company of their family members, and the bathing area should be well ventilated. The immersion time should not be too long (about 3-6 minutes) and when their heartbeat becomes faster or when they breathe harder during immersion, they should stand up slowly and rest in a well-ventilated area and return to immersion after recovery. They can take the bath in two to three rounds.

部分使用者(尤其是较为肥胖的使用者)浴后皮肤出现轻微刺痛感或出现小丘疹,均属排毒自然现象,可继续使用。

Some users (especially those who are very fat) will have slight tingling or small pimples on their skin after bath, which are all natural phenomena to excrete toxins and they can continue taking the bath.

5. 产妇生产时如有手术行为,待拆线后再进行药浴。

5. The lying-in women who have an operation during delivery should take the bath after taking out the stitches.

若无手术行为,可产后 3 天开始药浴。

If no operation is taken, they can take the medicated bath 3 days after delivery.

6. 体弱者在浸泡过程中可能出现头晕、心跳加快、恶心、全身无力等症状,一般属正常现象,严重的可以停止或用药。

6. Those who are weak may develop such symptoms as dizziness, heartbeat acceleration, sickness and general weakness during immersion, which are all normal phenomena, and they can stop the bathing or take medicine if the symptoms become severe.

体质越差越明显,随着不断地泡浴对体质进行调整,以上症状会逐渐消失。

The poorer the constitution is, the more evident the symptoms will be, and the above symptoms will gradually disappear as people continually take the bath to adjust the constitution.

7. 体虚、风寒重、体内毒素过多、湿毒偏重的人泡浴中,身体在药力作用下会将毒素或风寒排出体外,容易出现风疹、湿疹并伴有瘙痒等症状,属正常现象,一般 2 小时后消失。

7. People who are weak, or have severe wind cold, or have too many toxins or more damp-toxin inside the body will be likely to develop such symptoms as rubella and eczema combined with pruritus, which are all normal phenomena and will disappear 2 hours later. This is because these toxins and wind-cold are ejected out of the body under the action of medicine efficacy.

当有上述症状出现时只要坚持泡 1~3 个疗程症状即可消失。

As long as people insist on taking the bath for 1-3 courses of treatment when above-mentioned symptoms appear, the symptoms will disappear.

8. 手指与脚趾是通气的地方,所以泡瑶浴时注意应该露出手指。

8. Fingers and toes are where air is ventilated; therefore, people should make

their fingers out when taking Yao bath.

9. 皮肤有较大面积创口者禁浴。

9. Those who have larger wound on their skin should not take the bath.

10. 严重哮喘病、癫痫、恶性肿瘤、出血性疾病者禁浴。

10. Those who have serious asthma, epilepsy, malignant neoplasm and hemorrhagic diseases should not take the bath.

11. 过饥、过饱皆不宜泡浴。

11. Those who are too hungry and too full should not take the bath.

附:苗药浴

Attachment:Miao Medicated Bath

我国的传统医药学是各族人民的祖先创造的。

Our traditional medical science was created by ancestors of all peoples.

自有人类以来,各族人民的祖先们在生活生产中,在同大自然灾害的抗争中,在与各种野兽、毒虫伤害和疾病的斗争中,经历了从发现某种植物、动物、矿物能治疗某些疾病,到反复应用于人体验证,并付出了许多生命的试验中,创造总结出来了保护和维持各族人民身体健康及生存繁衍的民族传统文化和医药学知识。

Since the dawn of human beings, people from all the nations have experienced in life and production, in the struggle against natural disasters, in the fight against wild animals and poisonous insect injuries, and in the struggle against diseases from discovering the certain plants, animals and minerals can cure some diseases to applying them to human bodies for validation. In the process of experiment, they have lost a lot of lives and created and summarized the national tradition and culture and medical and pharmacological knowledge, protecting and maintaining the health, survival and reproduction of people from the nations.

由于各个民族所处的地理环境、自然生态、生产方式、生活习俗等不同,各民族所创造的民族医药学,从目前的基础理论、诊断方法、用药部位、加工炮制方法、治疗疾病等方面都各有所不同。

194

As the geographical environment, natural ecology, production mode and life custom of the nations are different, the medicines of the nations are different in the aspects of basic theories, diagnostic methods, medication positions, processing methods and disease treatment.

苗药浴应用的苗药是在苗族医药理论指导下, 由具有养生保健、防治疾病作用的原生态药材、原料药剂药品所组成。

The Miao medicine applied in Miao medicated bath is composed of the raw medicinal herbs and pharmaceutical chemicals that have functions of life cultivation, health care and disease prevention under the guidance of Miao medicine theories.

它是以苗医两纲(冷、热)、五经(风、热、冷、快、慢)、三十六症、七十二疾作为理论基础和诊治用药依据, 形成一个独立的民族医药学科。

Taking the 2 priciles (cold and hot), 5 classics (wind, hot, cold, fast and slow), 36 symptoms and 72 diseases of Miao medicine as the basic theory and the grounds for diagnosis and administration, Miao medicine forms an independent national medical discipline.

苗药浴是以苗药为基础, 具有疏通经络、活血化瘀、祛风散寒、清热解毒等作用。

On the basis of Miao medicine, Miao medicated bath has functions of dredging the meridians and collaterals, promoting blood circulation and removing blood stasis, expelling pathogenic wind and cold, clearing away heat and resolving toxins, etc.

参 考 文 献
References

[1] 蓝毓营. 庞桶药浴在瑶医防治疾病中的运用[J]. 广西中医药, 2014, 37(1):44-45.

[2] 唐生斌, 胡传贵. 瑶族民间药浴方药调查整理[J]. 中国民族医药杂志, 2000(3):26.

[3] 李彤, 闫国跃, 陈浪, 等. 瑶族庞桶药浴的应用研究[J]. 中国民间疗法, 2012, 20(3):45.

[4] 刘光海. 12 种基源相同的苗药侗药与中药的比较[J]. 中国民族医药杂志, 2009, 15(6):
24-26.

第三节　精油香熏浴
Chapter 3　Essential Oil Aromatherapy Bath

精油是从天然中草药和其他植物的花、叶、茎、根或果实中,通过水蒸气蒸馏法、挤压法、冷浸法或溶剂提取法提炼萃取的具有挥发性的芳香物质。

The essential oil is a volatile aromatic substance refined and extracted from natural Chinese herbal medicine, and flowers, leaves, stems and roots of plants, or fruits through steam distillation method, extrusion method, cold-maceration method or solvent extraction method.

精油里包含很多不同的成分,有的精油,例如玫瑰,可由 250 种以上不同的分子结合而成。

It contains many different components. Some essential oil, such as rose essential oil, is formed by combining more than 250 kinds of different molecules.

精油具有亲脂性,很容易溶在油脂中,因为精油的分子链通常比较短,这使得它们极易渗透于皮肤,通过皮下脂肪下丰富的毛细血管而进入体内。

The essential oil is lipophilic, and is very easy to dissolve in grease. Because the molecular chains of the essential oil are usually short, the molecular chains are very easy to penetrate into skin and enter the body through capillary vessels under subcutaneous fat.

精油是由一些很小的分子组成,这些高挥发性物质可由鼻腔黏膜组织吸收进入身体,将讯息直接送到脑部,通过大脑的边缘系统,调节情绪和身体的生理功能。

It is made up of very small molecules. These highly volatile substances can enter the body through mucosal tissue of the nasal cavity to directly transmit messages to the brain, so as to regulate emotional and physiological functions of the limbic system of the brain.

所以在芳香疗法中,精油可强化生理和心理的功能。

Therefore, in aromatherapy, the essential oil can strengthen physiological and psychological functions.

每一种植物精油都有一个化学结构来决定它的香味、色彩、流动性和系统运作的方式,这也使得每一种植物精油各有一套特殊的功能特质。

Every kind of plant essential oil has a chemical structure that determines its aroma, color, fluidity and systematic interaction mode, making every kind of plant essential oil also have a set of special function characteristics.

植物香熏浴是把精油通过泡浴的形式作用于人体,使得精油与人体在最大程度上得到接触,起到最好的效果,对促进身心健康有很好的功效。

Plant aromatherapy bath uses the essential oil to act on the human body in a form of bathing, so that the essential oil comes into contact with the human body to the largest degree, thereby performing the best effect. It has a good efficacy for promoting physical and mental health.

各种植物精油的功能各异,经常泡香熏浴可以促进血液循环、平衡内分泌、加快新陈代谢、防止肌肤老化、保湿滋润、提振精神、舒缓情绪、纤体瘦身等。

The functions of various plant essential oils are different. Frequent aromatherapy baths can promote blood circulation, balance endocrine, accelerate metabolism, prevent skin aging, keep moisture, enhance spirit, release the mood and lose weight, etc.

一、精油香熏浴的起源

Ⅰ. Origin of Essential Oil Aromatherapy Bath

关于精油的首批记载来自古代的印度、波斯和埃及。

The first record of essential oil comes from ancient India, Persia and Egypt.

希腊和罗马与东方各国进行了大量的芳香油和油膏贸易。

Greece and Rome made lots of trade with the eastern countries in essential oil and ointments.

这些产品很可能是用花朵、根和叶浸入脂油中而制出的萃取物。

These products are probably extracts made by immersing the flowers, roots and leaves in the tallow oil.

在大部分古代资料记载中,人们都是直接使用芳香植物或其树脂状产物。

In most ancient records, essential plants or their resinous products are used directly.

直到阿拉伯文化的黄金时代,才开发出蒸馏精油的技术。

It is not until the golden age of Arab culture that the technology of distilling essential oil was not developed.

阿拉伯人首先从发酵的糖中蒸馏出乙醇,从而提供了一种萃取精油的新溶剂,以代替可能已使用数千年的脂油。

The Arabs first distilled alcohol from the fermented sugar, thus providing a new solvent of extracting essential oil to replace the tallow oil that might have been used for thousands of years.

二、精油香熏浴的作用机制及功效

Ⅱ. Action Mechanism and Efficacy of Essential Oil Aromatherapy Bath

精油香熏浴可预防传染病,对抗细菌、病毒、真菌等,可预防感染及痉挛,并促进细胞的再生功能。

Essential oil aromatherapy bath has the functions of preventing infectious diseases, resisting bacteria, viruses and fungi, preventing infection, preventing convulsion and promoting cell regeneration.

而某些精油能促进荷尔蒙的分泌,让人体的生理及心理活动获得良好的发展。

However, some essential oils can promote secretion of hormones and make physiological and psychological activities develop well.

不同种类的精油还有各种不同的功效,对于一些疾病,也有舒缓和减轻症状的功能,配合药物的治疗,可以让疾病恢复得更快。

Different kinds of essential oils have different efficacies. They have functions of soothing and alleviating symptoms of some diseases, and can also accelerate recovery of the disease through cooperation with medical treatment.

并且在日常生活中使用,可以起到净化空气、消毒、杀菌的功效。

The essential oil used in daily life also has functions of purifying the air, sterilization and disinfection.

精油香熏浴对于内分泌、新陈代谢有很好的调节作用,对呼吸系统疾病、血液循环系统疾病、消化系统疾病、泌尿系统疾病、免疫系统疾病、妇科疾病、骨科疾病、皮肤科疾病、性病、精神类疾病、五官科疾病有很好的疗效。

It has good regulating effects on endocrine and metabolism, and has good curative effects on diseases of the respiratory system, blood circulatory system, digestive system, urological system and immune system, gynecological diseases, orthopaedic diseases, dermatologic disease, venereal diseases, mental diseases and sense-organs diseases.

精油香熏浴有以下主要功能:

Essential oil aromatherapy bath has the following functions:

1. 呼吸系统 植物精油分子通过鼻腔黏膜系统吸收刺激嗅觉神经,嗅觉神经将刺激传至大脑中枢,大脑产生兴奋,以加强呼吸道的免疫功能,起到抗病毒、发汗、解热、化痰等作用。

1. Respiratory system Plant essential oil molecules are absorbed through mucosal system of the nasal cavity and then stimulate the olfactory nerves, which then transmit stimulation to the cerebral center, making the cerebrum produce excitation. This will enhance the immune function of respiratory tract, and have functions of anti-virus, sweating, heat-relieving and phlegm elimination, etc.

2. 神经系统 通过亲和作用直接进入皮下,植物精油分子可直接刺激交感神经及副交感神经,起到镇静及催眠、兴奋提神、调整精神状态、抗忧郁、缓解心理压力、修复神经系统的作用,最终达到调节神经活动及内循环的目的。

2. Nervous system Directly entering the subcutaneous tissue through affinity, plant essential oil molecules can directly stimulate the sympathetic nerve and parasympathetic nerve, which plays roles in tranquilizing and hypnosis, excitation and mind refreshment, spirit condition adjustment, anti-depression, mental pressure alleviation and nervous system renovation, thus achieving the purpose of adjusting nervous activities and internal circulation.

3. 代谢系统 通过亲和作用植物精油分子迅速改善局部组织、细胞的生存环境,使其新陈代谢加快。

3. **Metabolic system** Under affinity interaction, plant essential oil molecules can rapidly improve the living environment of local tissues and cells, thus accelerating their metabolism.

又经体液交换进入血液和淋巴,促进了血液和淋巴循环,加快了人体的新陈代谢。

They also enter the blood and lymph through body fluid exchange, which promotes the circulation of blood and lymph and accelerates the metabolism of human body.

4. **循环系统** 加速血液、淋巴循环,降低血压。

4. **Circulatory system** Accelerating the circulation of blood and lymph and lowering blood pressure.

5. **皮肤系统** 具有杀菌、抗感染、愈合、除臭、镇静、驱虫、柔润细腻皮肤等作用。

5. **Dermal system** Having actions of disinfection, anti-infection, healing, deodorization, tranquilizing, parasite expulsion, moisturizing and softening the skin, etc.

6. **消化系统** 止痉挛、开胃、祛风、促进胆汁分泌、保肝等作用。

6. **Digestive system** Having actions of anti-spasm, appetite stimulation, dispelling wind, promoting choleresis, nourishing the liver, etc.

7. **免疫系统** 抗细菌、抗病毒、抗真菌、提高细胞防御、排毒、驱虫等作用。

7. **Immune system** Having actions of anti-bacterium, anti-virus, anti-fungal, cytophylaxis improvement, toxin elimination and parasite expulsion, etc.

8. **肌肉与骨骼系统** 抗炎性、抗风湿性、净化、舒缓肌肉组织、排毒等作用。

8. **Muscle skeletal system** Having actions of anti-inflammation, anti-rheumatism, purifying, muscular tissue soothing and toxin expulsion, etc.

9. **内分泌系统** 其所含有的仿雌激素与植物类固醇,可通过刺激肾上腺及甲状腺,达到降低血糖、降低血压、平衡各分泌系统平衡的作用。

9. **Endocrine system** The xenoestrogens and phytosterols contained in the essential oil can achieve the functions of lowering the blood sugar, lowering blood

pressure and balancing secretory systems through stimulating the adrenal gland and thyroid gland.

10. 女性生殖系统 抗痉挛、调经、催乳、调节乳汁分泌、影响荷尔蒙分泌、强化子宫等作用。

10. Female reproductive system　Having actions of anti-convulsion, menstruation regulation, lactescence adjustment, hormone secretion regulation and uterus strengthening, etc.

三、各种精油配方

Ⅲ. Formula of Different Essential Oils

1. 薰衣草 具有帮助睡眠、使人镇静、促进细胞再生、平衡皮脂分泌、治灼伤与晒伤的作用,可以改善湿疹、干癣和瘢痕。

1. Lavender　It has functions of improving sleep, tranquilizing, promoting cell regeneration, balancing sebum secretion, and curing scalds and sunburns. It can also improve the conditions of eczema, psoriasis and scar.

还可以缓解肌肉疼痛、痛经、头痛头晕,抗风湿、流行性感冒,治烧伤、创伤,降血压,驱虫等。

It also has functions of relieving muscular pain, algomenorrhea, headache and dizziness; anti-rheumatism, anti-influenza; burn and wound curing; blood pressure reduction and parasite expulsion, etc.

2. 玫瑰 具有保湿去皱,美白淡斑,淡化细纹,收敛毛孔,消除黑眼圈和妊娠纹,收缩微血管,促进细胞再生的作用。

2. Rose　It has functions of moisturizing and removing wrinkle, whitening and spot solution, fine wrinkle reduction, pore astringency, elimination of black eye and striae gravidarum, capillary contraction and cell regeneration promotion, etc.

还可以调节月经、不孕症,平衡内分泌,舒缓经前综合征,延缓更年期,抗菌、消毒等。

It also has functions of adjusting menstruation and infertility, balancing endocrine, relieving premenstrual syndrome, delaying climacterium, antibacterium, sterilization, etc.

3. 茉莉 具有保湿、改善敏感皮肤、淡化妊娠纹及瘢痕、增进皮肤弹性、助产、促乳汁分泌、调节呼吸、放松肌肉、平衡荷尔蒙、舒缓子宫痉挛的作用,还可以改善性冷淡及不孕症,延缓更年期。

3. Jasmine   It has the functions of moisturizing, improving sensitive skin, fading out the striae gravidarum and scar, and promoting skin elasticity. It can aid parturition, promote lactescence, adjust respiration, relax the muscles, balance hormone, relieve hysteron spasm, improve sexual apathy and infertility and delay climacterium.

4. 柠檬 具有美白淡斑、平衡油脂分泌、收敛毛孔、改善破裂微血管、软化皮肤的作用,还可治疗暗疮和扁平疣。

4. Lemon   It has functions of whitening and spot solution, balancing oil secretion, pore astringency, improving broken capillaries, softening skins and curing acnes and verruca plana.

5. 檀香 具有平衡干性湿疹及老化缺水的皮肤,使皮肤软化的作用,可以改善皮肤发痒、发炎、面部疱、疥和感染的伤口。

5. Sandalwood   It has functions of balancing the hydropenic skin with asteatotic eczema and aging as well as softening the skin. It can also improve itchiness, inflammation, acnes, scabies and infected wounds.

还可以治疗膀胱炎、胃胀气、腹泻、支气管炎等疾病。

It can also cure such diseases as cystitis, gaseous distention, diarrhoea and bronchitis.

6. 茶树 具有净化油性皮肤、抗菌、改善伤口感染化脓的作用,可应用于真菌引起的皮肤病,也可以治疗头皮过干与头皮屑。

6. Tea tree   It has the functions of purifying oil skin, antibacterium and improving wound infection and suppuration. It can be applied to the fungus-caused dermatosis and cure the overdry scalp and dandruff.

还可强化免疫系统,治疗牙周炎、哮喘、鼻炎、伤风感冒、瘙痒、生殖系统感染等疾病。

It can also strengthen the immune system, cure diseases like periodontitis, asthma, rhinitis, cold, pruritus, reproductive system infection.

7. 鼠尾草　具有促进细胞再生的作用,尤其有利于头皮部位毛发生长,能净化油腻的发质及头皮,有益于发炎和肿胀的皮肤恢复正常。

7. Salvia　It can promote cell regeneration and is beneficial to the hair growth in the scalp, and it can also purify the greasy hair and scalp and help the inflamed and swollen skin return to normal.

治疗月经过少、更年期综合征、食欲不振、便秘、瘫痪、水肿、肥胖症等疾病。

It can also cure diseases like hypomenorrhea, climacteric syndrome, poor appetite, constipation, paralysis, oedema and obesity, etc.

8. 天竺葵　具有平衡皮脂分泌的作用,对松垮、毛孔阻塞及油性皮肤有益,堪称一种全面性的洁肤油,能促进血液循环,使皮肤红润,能调节荷尔蒙分泌,治疗经前期综合征,能利尿消肿,以强化循环系统,达到降低血糖的作用。

8. Geranium　It can balance the sebum secretion, and is beneficial to pore block and oily skin. It is a comprehensive skin cleaning, which can promote blood circulation, make the skin red and moisturized, regulating hormone secretion, curing premenstrual syndrome, diuretic swelling, strengthening circulatory system and lowering the blood sugar.

9. 佛手柑　可以治疗湿疹、粉刺、静脉曲张、伤口、疱疹、头皮和皮肤的脂溢性皮炎等疾病。

9. Bergamot　It can cure diseases like eczema, acnes, varicosity, wounds, herpes, and seborrhoeic dermatitis of scalp and skin.

10. 尤加利　对疱疹有显著功效,对烫伤亦有帮助,预防细菌滋生,促进新陈代谢,可改善阻塞的皮肤,改善伤风感冒、咳嗽、鼻窦炎、偏头痛、淋病、糖尿病、风湿病、支气管炎,向肺部提供氧气。

10. Eucalyptus　It has remarkable effects on herpes and is also helpful to scalds. It can prevent bacteria breeding, promote metabolism, improve obstructed skin, improve the cold, cough, nasosinusitis, hemicrania, gonorrhoea, diabetes, rheumatism and bronchitis and provide oxygen to the lung.

11. 甜橙　具有保湿、美白淡斑、预防皱纹、淡化妊娠纹的作用,可以促进新陈代谢、排毒、健胃、利消化、刺激胆汁分泌、促进食欲、抗病毒、舒缓肌肉疼痛等。

11. Sweet orange It is effective in moisturizing, whitening and spot fading, prevention of wrinkles and fading out the striae gravidarum. It can promote metabolism, expel toxin, invigorate the stomach, facilitate digestion, stimulate bile secretion, promote appetite, resist virus, soothe muscular pain, etc.

12. 迷迭香 具有紧实松垮皮肤、减轻充血浮肿的作用。

12. Rosemary It is effective in tightening the loose skin and reducing hyperemia and swelling.

对头皮失调特别有帮助,改善头皮屑并刺激毛发生长。

It is especially helpful in treating scalp disorders. It can resolve dandruff and stimulate hair growth.

刺激免疫系统,改善腹泻、呼吸道疾病、肥胖、痛经、泌尿系统疾病、肌肉疼痛等。

It can stimulate the immune system and improve diarrhea, respiratory diseases, obesity, dysmenorrhea, urinary system diseases, muscular pain, etc.

13. 薄荷 具有净化皮肤、平衡油脂分泌的作用。

13. Peppermint It is effective in purifying the skin and balancing grease secretion.

治疗暗疮粉刺,收缩微细血管,舒缓发炎红肿。

It treats acnes, contracts blood capillaries and relieves inflammatory redness and swelling.

改善消化系统,可治疗感冒、头痛、牙疼、风湿痛、肌肉酸痛等。

It improves the digestive system and treats cold, headache, toothache, rheumatic pain, muscular soreness, etc.

四、精油香熏浴使用方法

Ⅳ. Method of Administration for Essential Oil Aromatherapy Bath

1. 浸浴 先将 6~8 滴的精油滴入一汤匙的牛奶或酒精中(介质,便于精油与水混合),再加入 30~40℃的热水中,浸泡 20 分钟。

1. Immersion bath　Firstly drop 6-8 drops of essential oil into a spoonful of milk or alcohol(a medium, being convenient for mixing the essential oil with water), then put it into hot water of 30-40℃, immersing for 20 minutes.

2. 淋浴　在沐浴液中加入 1~2 滴的精油。

2. Shower　1-2 drops of essential oil are added to bath water.

3. 足浴　可用于治疗脚气、灰指甲、脚扭伤、高血压等。也可以用于放松情绪、改善循环、足部皮肤的保养等。

3. Foot bath　It can be used for treating beriberi, tinea unguium, foot spraining, hypertension, etc. It can also be used for relaxing the mood, improving the circulation, maintaining foot skin, etc.

4. 手浴　可用于治疗冻疮、灰指甲及手部皮肤的保养等。

4. Hand bath　It can be used for treating chilblain, tinea unguium, hand skin care, etc.

5. 盆浴　将 1~2 滴的精油滴入牛奶中搅匀,倒入清水中用手搅拌一下,避免精油浮在水面上,刺激黏膜。

5. Bath in a tub　1-2 drops of essential oil are added to milk, mixed well and poured into clean water, and the mixture is stirred by hand to avoid the essential oil from floating on the water and stimulating mucosa.

适用于男女阴部、肛门疾病,如女性阴道炎、外阴部瘙痒、男性阴囊炎、湿疹、痔疮等,也可用于阴部清洁保健。

It applies to the diseases of the pudenda and anus of men and women, such as female vaginitis, pruritus vulvae, male scrotitis, eczema and hemorrhoid, and also applies to vaginal cleaning and health care.

6. 敷盖法　将精油用牛奶稀释倒入清水中,搅拌均匀后,将毛巾浸泡、拧干,敷于患部。

6. Application method　The essential oil is diluted with milk and then poured into clean water to make a mixture by well stirring. The towel is immersed with the mixture, wrung out and applied to the affected part.

可针对肌肉酸痛、神经痛、关节痛、局部发炎、头痛、偏头痛等。

It can be applied to muscular soreness, neuralgia, arthralgia, local inflammation, headache, migraine, etc.

可改善关节扭伤、发炎、感冒、发热、头痛及敏感皮肤,油性、暗疮性皮肤,毛孔粗大等症状。

It can improve the symptoms such as joint sprain, inflammation, cold, fever, headache, sensitive skin, oily skin, acne-prone skin, coarse pores, etc.

温敷一般在美容按摩前,针对干性、缺水性肌肤。

Warm compress is normally applied to the dry and dehydrated skin before facial beauty massage.

7. 护发 用1~2滴精油加入洗发精或洗发水中,于头部按摩数分钟后冲洗。

7. Hair care 1-2 drops of essential oil are added to the shampoo or liquid shampoo, with which the head is massaged for a few minutes, and it is washed afterwards.

适用于头屑、油性发质、易脱发、发质损伤者。

It applies to the patients with dandruff, oily hair, alopecia and damaged hair.

五、精油香熏浴使用的注意事项

Ⅴ. Precautions for Use of Essential Oil Aromatherapy Bath

1. 精油通常不能直接涂抹于皮肤上,要经过基础油稀释过才能用在皮肤上。

1. The essential oil should not be smeared onto the skin directly, and it can only be smeared onto the skin after dilution with the base oil.

2. 精油具有较强的挥发性,必须用深色的遮光瓶包装,用完后应及时将盖子盖上。

2. The essential oil has strong volatility, and must be packed by a dark sunscreen bottle and should be covered with a lid in time after being used.

保存在避光、通风、干燥的地方。

The essential oil should be kept in light-resistant, ventilating and dry places.

避免使用塑料用品。

Using of plastic articles should be avoided.

3. 柑橘类精油具有光敏性,如柠檬、甜橙,应避免阳光照射,不可在白天使用。

3. The citrus essential oil light-sensitive, for example, lemons and oranges should be avoided being exposed in the sun and not be used during the daytime.

薄荷在夜间不可使用。

The peppermint should not be used during the night.

4. 一种单方精油不可连续使用超过 3 个月,要适当调换品种。

4. One kind of pure essential oil should not be used for more than three successive months and the varieties of essential oil should be changed appropriately.

5. 病人及孕妇、儿童等使用精油时更要注意,应先了解精油的禁忌,如明确说明病人、孕妇及儿童不能使用的,就一定不能使用。

5. More attention should be paid when the patients, pregnant women and children use the essential oil. The contraindications of essential oil should be learnt first and it cannot be used when there is a specific instruction of contraindication to patients, pregnant women and children.

6. 单方精油用于泡澡、泡手、泡脚时,要用牛奶稀释,再倒入清水中搅拌,避免灼伤肌肤。

6. When one kind of pure essential oil is used individually for bathing and soaking hands and feet, the essential oil should be first diluted with milk and then poured into clean water to avoid scalding the skin.

不可将单方精油直接倒入水中稀释。

Do not pour the pure essential oil directly into the water to dilute.

参 考 文 献
References

[1] 吴宇峰,李利荣,时庭锐,等. 香薰植物精油主要成分的气相色谱/质谱分析[J]. 中国

卫生检验杂志,2007,17(1):77-78.

[2] 杜红,宫小勇,高阿妮,等.药浴联合香薰护理提高宫颈癌术后患者生活质量的护理体会[J].中医药导报,2016,22(20):113-115.

第四节 中药药浴
Chapter 4 Chinese Medicated Bath

中药药浴系将中草药煎成汤液,稀释后沐浴全身或浸泡局部,利用水温本身对皮肤、经络、穴位的刺激和药物的透皮吸收作用,以通行经络血脉,内达脏腑,由表及里,从而产生治疗保健作用的一种中医传统外治方法,自古以来一直受到医学界的重视。

The Chinese medicated bath is a traditional external therapy of Chinese medicine, in which Chinese herbs are decocted with water into decoction which is then diluted to wash over the whole body or immerse certain body parts. It is using the stimulation of the water temperature itself to the skin, meridians, collaterals and acupoints and the transdermal absorption of the medicine to go through meridians, collaterals and blood vessels into zang-fu organs, from the exterior to the interior, thereby playing a therapeutic and health care function. It is a method that has drawn attention from the medical field since ancient times.

药浴在中国有悠久的历史,据载自周朝开始就流行用中药佩兰煎的药水泡浴,名为香汤浴。

The medicated bath has had several thousand years of history in China, and as recorded, the fragrant decoction bath has become popular since the Zhou dynasty. The so-called fragrant decoction is the medicinal liquid decocted from the herba eupatorii.

《黄帝内经》中就有"其受外邪者,渍形以为汗"的记载。

It is recorded in the *Inner Canon of Huangdi* that "a patient with invasion of exogenous pathogens can be given an immersion of the body with hot water to induce sweating".

晋、南北、隋唐时期,临床医学发展迅速,药浴被广泛地应用到临床各科。

During the Jin, Southern & Northern and Sui & Tang dynasties when clinical medicine had developed rapidly, the medicated bath was widely applied to various clinical departments.

宋、金、元、明时期,药浴的方药不断增多,应用范围逐渐扩大,药浴成为一种常用的治疗方法。

During the Song, Jin, Yuan and Ming dynasties when prescriptions for medicated bath continuously had increased and application scope thereof was extended gradually, the medicated bath became a common treatment method.

到了清朝,药浴发展到了鼎盛阶段,清代名医辈出,名著相继刊出。

By the Qing dynasty, the medicated bath has reached its peak, therefore well-known doctors came forth in large numbers and famous books were published successively.

随着《急救广生集》《理瀹骈文》等中医药外治专著的出现,中药药浴疗法已进入比较成熟和完善的阶段。

With the emergence of such monographs about external therapy of the Chinese medicine as *Collection of First Aid for Human Beings* and the *Rhymed Discourse for Topical Remedies*, the Chinese medicated bath therapy has entered a relatively mature and perfect stage.

一、药浴治疗的理论基础

I. Theoretical Basis of Medicated Bath Therapy

源自传统医学理论背景下的药浴疗法,中医学不乏对其有着详细的理论阐述,而现代医学也对外治法作用机制进行了深入的探究。

For the medicated bath therapy in the context of traditional medicine theory, there has been no lack of detailed theoretical elaboration on it, while in modern medicine there also has been a further investigation on the function mechanisms of external treatment.

（一）中医学对药浴治疗的理论基础

（I）Theoretical Basis of Medicated Bath Therapy in TCM

我国医学现存最早的外治法专著为清代医家吴尚先的《理瀹骈文》,本书原名《外治医说》,刊于 1870 年。

The earliest existing monograph of TCM external treatment is the *Rhymed Discourse for Topical Remedies* written by Wu Shangxian at the Qing dynasty, the original name of which is the *Medicine Theory of External Therapy* published in 1870.

吴尚先研究中医外治法数十年,积累了丰富的实践经验,后历时二十载,易稿十余次著成《理瀹骈文》,该书对中医外治法的总结与发展作出了重大贡献,《理瀹骈文》被后人尊称为"外治之宗"。

Having studied the external treatment of TCM for decades, Wu Shangxian had accumulated rich practical experience, and then finally finished the *Rhymed Discourse for Topical Remedies*, but it took a period of 20 years to revise the manuscript for more than 10 times. This book had made great contributions to the summarization and development of the external treatment of TCM and was later known as the "master of external treatment".

吴尚先在《理瀹骈文·略言》中开宗明义提出颇有哲理的重要观点:"外治之理,即内治之理,外治之药亦即内治之药,所异者法耳。医理药性无二,而法则神奇变换。"即外治与内治一样均是以中医基本理论为指导,明阴阳五行,识脏腑经络,辨寒热虚实,分标本缓急等。

In the *Outline of Rhymed Discourse for Topical Remedies*, Wu came straight to the philosophical points: "The principle of external treatment is equal to that of internal treatment, and the medicine of external treatment is also equal to that of internal treatment, the difference lies only in therapy. There are no difference in principle of medical science and nature of medicine, and it is the therapy that varies magically." Namely, both the external treatment and the internal treatment are guided by the theoretical basis of TCM, that is, understanding the yin-yang and five elements, knowing the zang-fu organs, meridians and collaterals, differentiating the cold from the hot and deficiency from excess and distinguishing between root cause and symptoms and the chronic from the acute.

外治与内治在医理与药性上并没有区别,所异者,法耳,只是在方法上有所不同,所异者只是饮之内与施之外,这些外治与内治机制统一的原则,一直有效地指导着临床实践。

There is no difference between the external treatment and the internal treatment in principle of medical science and nature of medicine, the difference lies in therapy, that is, oral administration and external application. The uniform principle of external treatment and internal treatment has always been effective in guiding the clinical practices.

在这一理论指导下,药浴治疗的遣方用药与内服法无异,且获得了良好的临床疗效。

Under the guidance of this theory, the principles of prescription and medication for medicated bath is the same as those for internal therapy and the medicated bath has also achieved good clinical effects.

(二) 现代医学对外治法治疗的理论基础

(Ⅱ) Theoretical Basis of External Treatment in Modern Medicine

现代研究表明,药浴液中的药物有效成分可通过皮肤黏膜的吸收、扩散、辐射等途径进入体内。

Modern researches indicate that the active ingredients of medicated bath can enter the human body through absorption, diffusion and radiation of the skin mucous membrane.

皮肤是人体最大的器官,除保护作用外,还具有吸收、渗透、感觉、分泌、排泄等多种功能,在人体的生理病理方面发挥着重要的作用。

Skin is the largest organ of human body. Besides protection, it also has multifunctions like absorption, penetration, feeling, secretion and excretion, etc., and plays an important function in physiology and pathology.

药物经皮吸收,途径有三:通过渗透角质层细胞膜,入其胞内;大分子及水溶性物质通过毛孔、汗孔被吸收;少量还可通过表面细胞间隙渗透进入真皮。

The medicine is absorbed through the skin in three ways:Some medicine enters the cell through permeation into the cuticle cytomembrane;macromolecules and water soluble substances are absorbed through pores;another small amount of medicine can penetrate into the skin through the space between surface cells.

药物经皮吸收避免口服引起的首过效应、胃肠反应等。

Absorption of the medicine through skin can avoid the first pass effect and gastrointestinal reaction caused by oral administration.

皮肤分布的大量脊、自主神经末梢及特殊感受器,在刺激作用下可以影响附近的接收器,从而调节神经、体液、循环功能,改善相应各组织器官的活动以增强机体的抗病和修复能力。

A great number of spinal and autonomic nerve terminals and special sensory receptors in the skin can influence the nearby receptors under stimulation, so that the neurological, humoral and circulatory functions are regulated and the activities of the corresponding tissues and organs are improved to enhance the disease resistance and recovery capability.

此外,皮肤的分泌、排泄、代谢功能参与机体对尿酸、尿素及一些无机盐等代谢产物的排泄,同时也参与对病体毒素及堆积代谢废物的排除,即中医所谓"透邪外出"。

In addition, the secretion, excretion and metabolism of skin participate in the excretion of uric acid, urea and some inorganic salts from the body, and also participate in the removal of the toxins and accumulated metabolic wastes from the sick body, that is, so called expelling pathogenic factors from the interior in TCM.

药浴疗法正是利用了这些生理功能来治疗疾病。

The medicated bath therapy just takes advantages of these physiological functions to cure diseases.

二、药浴的操作技术

Ⅱ. Operation Techniques of Medicated Bath

(一) 操作前准备

(Ⅰ) Preparation before Operation

1.**药物准备**　中药饮片的使用应符合《中华人民共和国药典》的规定。

1. Medicine Preparation　The CMM decoction pieces should be used in accordance with the *Pharmacopoeia of the People's Republic of China*.

中药药液的煎煮场地应符合《医疗机构中药煎药室管理规范》的规定。

The site for decocting Chinese medicine should conform to the *Specification for Management of Traditional Chinese Medicine Decoction Room*.

2.**器具选择**　宜选择规格:长 × 宽 × 高为 1.5m×0.6m×0.8m 的木质或竹质浴桶。

2. Appliance Selection   Preferred specification：1.5m length × 0.6m width × 0.8m height，wooden or bamboo bath bucket.

3. 环境要求　配备相对独立的接待区、更衣区、休息区、浴区、中药煎液制备区。

3. Environmental Requirements   Relatively independent reception area，dressing area，resting area，bath area and Chinese traditional medicine decoction preparing area should be provided.

配备急救人员、急救设备及药品。

The first aider，first aid equipment and medicines should be provided.

配有水温调节装置及温度测量设备。

The water temperature regulator and the temperature measuring equipment should be provided.

环境宜安静，避免噪音。

The environment should be quiet and free of noise.

室内干净、舒适、无异味，有防滑设施与防跌倒标志，配备通风设施，保持房间空气流通，光线柔和，光照充足。

The room should be clean，comfortable and free of unpleasant smell，and be provided with anti-slip facilities，falls-prevention signs and ventilation facilities to keep the room ventilated，with a soft light and sufficient illumination.

室内温度（32 ± 3）℃，室内湿度 60% ± 10%。

The room temperature is（32 ± 3）℃，and the room humidity is 60%±10%.

4. 消毒　应符合《GB15982—2012 医院消毒卫生标准》（现行）的规定。

4. Sterilization   It should conform to the *GB15982—2012 Hygienic Standard for Disinfection in Hospitals*（Current Standard）.

5. 施术前评估　由专业培训人员评估。

5. Preoperative Assessment   Professionally trained workers perform assessment.

施术前应根据受术者一般情况、药浴适应证及禁忌证进行适应性评估。

Adaptability assessment should be performed before operation based on the general conditions of the patients, medicated bath indications and contraindications.

告知受术者药浴注意事项。

The patients should be notified of precautions for medicated bath.

(二) 施术方法

(Ⅱ) Operation Methods

1. 根据评估结果及保健治疗需要, 预(配)制中药浴液。

1. Liquid for medicated bath is prepared according to the assessment results and the needs for health care treatment.

2. 受术者中药饮片用量如下:

2. Dosage of CMM decoction pieces for acceptor is as follows:

(1) 患者人群中药饮片最小用量 260g。

(1) For the patient group, the minimum dosage of the CMM decoction pieces is 260g.

(2) 亚健康人群中药饮片最小用量 230g。

(2) For sub-healthy group, the minimum dosage of the CMM decoction pieces is 230g.

(3) 健康人群中药饮片最小用量 200g。

(3) For healthy group, the minimum dosage of the CMM decoction pieces is 200g.

3. 受术时间应在餐后 1~2 小时内进行。

3. Operation time: The operation should be performed within 1-2 hours after the meal.

4. 浴桶内注入 0.4m 深的清水, 将预制好的中药煎液缓缓倒入浴桶内调和, 制备中药浴液。

4. Clean water is added into the bath bucket with a depth of 0.4m, and the prepared Chinese traditional medicine decoction is slowly poured into the bath bucket to prepare the compounding liquid for medicated bath.

5. 根据受术者需求初始水温设定在(40±2)℃。

5. The initial water temperature is set to $(40 \pm 2)℃$ according to the requirement of the acceptor.

6. 协助受术者进入浴桶。

6. The acceptor is assisted in entering the bath bucket.

7. 受术者可自行调节水温。

7. The acceptor can adjust the water temperature himself/herself.

8. 浴前先淋浴洁身。

8. Before entering the bath bucket, the acceptor should take a shower bath to clean the body.

9. 取坐位或半卧位泡浴,液面颈部以下,以舒适为宜。

9. The acceptor takes a sitting or semi-reclining position to take a bath comfortably, with the level of the liquid below the neck.

10. 每次泡浴时间 10~30 分钟。

10. Bath time is 10~30 minutes each time.

11. 结束时,宜缓慢起身,离开浴器(浴区),擦干全身。

11. After finishing the medicated bath, the acceptor should slowly get up, leave the bath(bath area) and wipe-dry the whole body.

12. 宜在尊重患者隐私和保证患者安全的前提下适度巡视。

12. It is preferred that the doctor should visit the acceptor appropriately on the premises of respecting the privacy and ensuring the safety of the patient.

13. 频次及疗程:隔日 1 次,3 周一疗程。

13. Frequency and Course of Treatment:The medicated bath should be taken once every other day, and 3 weeks make a course.

(三) 施术后处理

(Ⅲ) Processing after Operation

药浴后,温水冲洗。

After finishing the medicated bath, the acceptor should wash the body with warm water.

药浴后,应休息 5~10 分钟,无不适症状,方可离开。

After the medicated bath, the acceptor needs a rest for 5-10 minutes, and cannot leave until he/she has no uncomfortable symptom.

药浴后，皮肤多会发红，属正常反应。

After the medicated bath, the skin may turn red in most cases, which is a normal reaction.

如出现过敏症状，及时对症处理。

If an allergic symptom occurs, specific treatment should be performed accordingly in time.

药浴后，应注意保暖，避免感受风寒。

After the medicated bath, the acceptor should keep warm to avoid catching cold.

药浴后，宜适量补充水分和热量。

After the medicated bath, the acceptor should take a moderate amount of water and energy.

三、临床应用

Ⅲ. Clinical Application

（一）适应证

（Ⅰ）Indications

1. 内科　感冒、失眠、慢性肾功能不全、风湿病、高脂血症、高血压、糖尿病周围神经病变等。

1. In Internal Medicine　Cold, insomnia, chronic renal insufficiency, rheumatism, hyperlipemia, hypertension, diabetic peripheral neuropathy, etc.

2. 骨伤科　颈椎病、肩周炎、腰椎间盘突出症、骨性关节炎、坐骨神经痛、落枕、急性腰扭伤（48 小时后）等。

2. In Osteology and Traumatology　Cervical spondylosis, scapulohumeral periarthritis, prolapse of lumber intervertebral disc, osteoarthritis, sciatica, stiff neck, acute lumbar muscle sprain（after 48 hours）, etc.

3. 妇科　痛经、月经不调等。

3. In Gynecology　Dysmenorrhea, irregular menstruation, etc.

4. **儿科**　小儿外感发热、新生儿黄疸、小儿腹泻等。

4. In Pediatrics　Infantile exogenous fever, neonatal jaundice, infantile diarrhea, etc.

5. **皮肤科**　银屑病、皮炎、皮肤瘙痒、带状疱疹等。

5. In Dermatology　Psoriasis, dermatitis, cutaneous pruritus, herpes zoster, etc.

（二）处方示例

（Ⅱ）Prescription Examples

1. **小儿外感发热**

1. Infantile Exogenous Fever

（1）外感风寒发热：荆芥、桂枝、麻黄、防风、艾叶、生姜。

（1）Fever caused by exogenous cold: Fineleaf schizonepeta herb, cassia twig, Chinese ephedrine, divaricate saposhnikovia root, argy wormwood leaves and fresh ginger.

（2）外感风热发热：柴胡、青蒿、薄荷、连翘、荆芥、炒牛蒡子、川芎。

（2）Fever caused by exogenous wind-heat: Chinese thorowax root, sweet wormwood herb, peppermint, weeping forsythia capsule, fineleaf schizonepeta herb, stir-baked great burdock achene and Sichuan lovage rhizome.

（3）外感暑湿发热：青蒿、白矾、藿香、柴胡、薄荷、石膏、连翘、荆芥、蝉蜕。

（3）Fever caused by exogenous summerheat-dampness: Sweet wormwood herb, alum, wrinkled giant hyssop, Chinese thorowax root, peppermint, gypsum, weeping forsythia capsule, fineleaf schizonepeta herb and cicada slough.

2. **失眠**

2. Insomnia

（1）肝郁化火证：合欢皮、柴胡、菊花、决明子。

（1）Syndrome of liver depression transforming into fire: Silktree albizia bark, Chinese thorowax root, chrysanthemum flower and Cassia occidentalis.

（2）痰热内扰证：黄芩、竹茹、陈皮、茯苓皮。

（2）Syndrome of phlegm-heat attacking internally: Baical skullcap root, bamboo shavings, dried tangerine peel and Indian bread peel.

（3）阴虚火旺证：黄柏、茯神、麦冬、沙参。

（3）Syndrome of hyperactivity of fire due to yin deficiency: Amur cork-tree, poria with hostwood, dwarf lilyturf tuber and ladybell.

（4）心脾两虚证：党参、酸枣仁、茯苓、五味子。

（4）Syndrome of deficiency of both heart and spleen: Tangshen, spina date seed, Indian bread and five flavours.

（5）心虚胆怯证：柏子仁、夜交藤、龙骨、牡蛎。

（5）Syndrome of timidity due to deficiency of heart qi: Chinese arborvitae kernel, tuber fleeceflower stem, bone fossil of big mammals and oyster shell.

3. 骨性关节炎

3. Osteoarthritis

（1）寒湿痹阻证：杜仲、狗脊、仙茅、锁阳、淫羊藿、羌活、独活、防风。

（1）Syndrome of cold-damp obstruction: Eucommia bark, cibot rhizoma, common curculigo rhizome, songaria cynomorium herb, epimedium herb, incised notopterygium rhizome and root, doubleteeth pubescent angelica root and divaricate saposhnikovia root.

（2）湿热痹阻证：薏苡仁、泽泻、茯苓、羌活、独活、黄芩、秦艽、通草。

（2）Syndrome of damp-heat obstruction: Coix seed, oriental waterplantain rhizome, Indian bread, incised notopterygium rhizome and root, doubleteeth pubescent angelica root, baical skullcap root, largeleaf gentian root and ricepaperplant pith.

（3）肝肾亏虚证：桑寄生、淫羊藿、枸杞、附子、狗脊、牛膝、熟地黄。

（3）Syndrome of deficiency of both liver and kidney: Parasite scurrula, epimedium herb, barbary wolfberry fruit, prepared common monkshood branched root, cibot rhizoma, twotoothed achyranthes root and prepared rehmannia root.

（三）禁忌证

（Ⅲ）Contraindications

1. 女性月经期禁用。

1. It is prohibited for women during menstrual period.

2. 不明原因疼痛、高热者禁用。

2. It is prohibited for those with unknown pains or high fever.

3. 患有严重高血压(血压≥160/100mmHg)或低血压(血压≤90/60mmHg)者禁用。

3. It is prohibited for patients with severe hypertension(blood pressure≥160/100 mmHg) or hypotension(blood pressure≤90/60 mmHg).

4. 重度精神性疾病、癫痫及抽搐等处于发作期,神经官能症、癔症神经功能紊乱及不能合作者禁用。

4. It is prohibited for patients with severe psychiosis, epilepsy and hyperspasmia in the attacking stage, neurosis, hysteria and nerve function disorder and those who cannot provide cooperation.

5. 有皮下血管瘤、不明原因肿块及局部水疱者禁用。

5. It is prohibited for those with subcutaneous angioma, unknown lump and local blister.

6. 大范围感染性病灶并已化脓破溃、感染及皮肤有开放性创口者禁用。

6. It is prohibited for patients with extensive festered, ulcerated and infected lesions, or with open wound on skin.

7. 软组织损伤者48小时内禁用。

7. It is prohibited for those with soft tissue injury within 48 hours.

8. 严重心肺功能不全或低下者禁用。

8. It is prohibited for patients with severe cardiopulmonary insufficiency or hypofunction.

(四) 注意事项

(Ⅳ) Precautions

1. 施术前应向受术者说明治疗的特点和治疗时可能出现的情况。

1. Before operation, the acceptor should be informed of treatment characteristics and situations possible to occur during treatment.

2. 体质虚弱及初次接受药浴者,药浴时间宜短。

2. The time of taking the medicated bath should be short for those with weak constitution and for those who take the medicated bath for the first time.

3. 饮酒、大量出汗、过度劳累后慎用。

3. Those who have drunk, sweated excessively or overworked should take the medicated bath with caution.

4. 皮肤过敏、破损者慎用。

4. Those with skin allergy or injury should take the medicated bath with caution.

5. 有传染性疾病者,应做好消毒及隔离工作。

5. Those with infectious diseases should be sterilized and isolated.

6. 高龄、孕妇、温度感应迟缓、局部麻木无知觉、语言障碍、认知障碍及运动功能障碍者慎用或专人全程陪护。

6. Pregnant women and those with advanced age, insensitivity to temperature, local numbness, speech disorder, cognitive disorder and dyskinesia should take the medicated bath with caution or with a special companion for the whole course.

7. 有出血倾向疾病及凝血功能异常者慎用。

7. Those with hemorrhagic tendency and coagulopathy should take the medicated bath with caution.

8. 泡浴过程中不应使用沐浴液等日化产品。

8. Household chemicals such as bath foam should not be used in the medicated bath.

(五) 意外的处理方法

(V) Treatment for Accidents

1. 头晕　如有头晕甚至意识障碍发生,应立即停止药浴治疗,使患者尽快离开潮湿闷热环境,将患者安全地置于通风处。

1. Dizziness　In case of dizziness or even disturbance of consciousness, stop medicated bath treatment immediately, take the patient away from the muggy environment and safely put him/her in a well-ventilated place.

让患者平卧,检查生命体征,视患者情况进一步检查急救或观察病情变化。

Let the patient lie on the back to be checked for vital signs and according to the situations of the patient, perform further checks or first aid, or observe disease development.

2. 溺水的处理 使患者尽快离开水中,令其平卧,检查生命体征,予心肺复苏支持,寻求急诊医师帮助。

2. Drowning Take the patient out of the water as soon as possible, and let him/her lie on the back to be checked for vital signs, give cardio-pulmonary resuscitation and seek help from emergency physicians.

3. 意外摔倒 询问或检查摔伤患处,判断创伤程度,简单处理患处,使患者安全离开药浴治疗区,避免二次创伤,对症处置并积极检查创伤病情以排除骨折、心脑血管疾病等。

3. Accidental falls Inquire or check fall damage, assess the severity of the damage, simply handle the injured part, take the patient away from the medicated bath therapy area to avoid further injury, perform specific treatment accordingly, and check injury conditions to exclude fracture, cardiovascular and cerebrovascular diseases, etc.

参 考 文 献
References

[1] 彭方雄. 浅谈吴师机"外治之理""外治之药"论[J]. 时珍国医国药,2001,12(3):239.
[2] 吴师机. 理瀹骈文[M]. 北京:人民卫生出版社,1984.
[3] 孙秀娟,周春祥. 药浴疗法作用机理探析[J]. 江西中医学院学报,2007,19(5):25-26.

第五节 温 泉 浴
Section 5 Hot Spring Bath

我国是世界上最早利用温泉治病的国家之一。

China is one of the first countries to use hot spring bath to treat diseases.

陕西临潼华清池温泉,早在两千多年以前就已开始用以治病,被称为"自然之经方,天地之元医"。

The hot spring of Huaqing Hot Spring in Lintong County, Shaanxi Province has been used to treat diseases since 2 000 years ago, which is referred to as "the classical prescription of nature and the fundamental therapy of the universe".

近年来,由于"现代康复医学"的迅速发展,温泉的康复作用越来越被相关专业的学者、医生所重视与应用。

In recent years, with the rapid development of "modern rehabilitation medicine", the rehabilitation effect of hot spring bath has gained increasing attention and application from the relevant professional scholars and doctors.

温泉若要具有治病和保健功能,一定要满足以下条件:

For the healing and health care functions, the hot spring must meet the following requirements:

①含有一定浓度的矿物质,每升水中含有固体成分在 1g 以上。

① It must have a certain concentration of minerals and there should be more than 1g of solid constituents per litre of hot spring water.

②含有一定量的气体,如二氧化碳、硫化氢、氡等。

② It must contain a certain amount of gas, such as CO_2, H_2S, Rn, etc.

③含有一定的微量元素,如铁、碘、溴、氟等。

③ It must contain a certain amount of trace elements, such as Fe, I, Br, F, etc.

只有具备了以上条件的温泉,才称得上是有保健和治疗功能的医疗矿泉。

Only by meeting the above conditions can hot spring be referred to as the medicinal spring with health care and healing functions.

也只有了解了温泉所具有的理化成分和特性,才能确定其保健治疗的适应证、禁忌证及具体的应用方法。

Also, only by understanding the physical-chemical compositions and characteristics of the hot spring can the indications and contraindications of health care and healing as well as its specific application methods be determined.

一、温泉浴治疗的理论基础

Ⅰ. Theoretical Basis of Hot Spring Bath Treatment

人们现已发现,温泉之所以有治病保健的疗效,是因为泉水对人体有非特异性和特异性两方面的作用。

It is found that the hot spring has the healing and health care functions, this is because the spring water has both non-specific and specific effects on human body.

所谓温泉的非特异性是指温泉水温、水压等对人体的物理作用。

The so-called non-specificity of the hot spring refers to the physical effect of water temperature and water pressure of the hot spring on the human body.

比如温热(一般在 25℃以上)的泉水,可使毛细血管扩张,促进血液循环;而水的机械浮力与静水压力作用,则可起到按摩、收敛、消肿、止痛效能。

For example, hot spring water (generally above 25℃) will dilate the blood capillary and promote blood circulation; and the mechanical buoyancy and hydrostatic pressure of water will have the effects of massage, convergence, apocatastasis and analgesia.

温泉的特异性作用则是指泉水中矿物质的化学作用。

The specific effect of the hot spring refers to the chemical effect of minerals in spring water.

据化验,大多数温泉水中都有一种可溶性元素——锗,有机锗具有抗癌作用。

According to the test, most of hot spring water contains a kind of soluble element-Ge, and organic germanium has the anti-cancer effect.

温泉中还含有硅、铂、锰、锌、碘、硒及碳酸盐、硫酸盐、硫、铅、铁、氟、硼等矿物质,对防病治病均有一定效果。

The hot spring also contains Si, Pt, Mn, Zn, I, Se and minerals such as carbonate, sulphate, S, Pb, Fe, F and B, which all have a certain effect in preventing and curing diseases.

从现代医学角度讲,有效成分及矿物质经透皮吸收渗入人体发挥积极正面的生物作用。从中医角度讲,水温本身对皮肤、经络、穴位的刺激作用,使得经络血脉通畅,祛邪扶正,从而产生治疗保健作用。

From the perspective of modern medicine, effective components and minerals penetrating into the human body through the skin can positively play a biological action. From the perspective of TCM, water temperature itself has stimulatory effect on skin, meridians, collaterals and acupoints, which will make meridians, collaterals and blood vessels unobstructed, and strengthen healthy qi to eliminate pathogens, thus bringing healing and health care effects.

（一）温度的刺激作用

（Ⅰ）Temperature Stimulation

温度不同,保健效果不一样。

Health care effects vary with temperatures.

比如,水温在 30~40℃时,可调节神经系统的兴奋、抑制过程,对轻度冠心病、早期高血压、自主神经功能紊乱、各种慢性炎症、关节疾病及皮肤病等有治疗效果。

For example, with water temperature of 30-40℃, the processes of excitation and inhibition of neural systems can be adjusted, and mild coronary heart disease, early hypertension, autonomic nervous system functional disturbance, various chronic inflammations, joint disease, skin disease and others can be treated.

水温在低于 34℃时,可以反射性地提高交感神经兴奋性,经常洗浴可提高机体对寒冷的应激适应能力,有增强体质、预防疾病的保健作用。

With water temperature below 34℃, the excitability of sympathetic nerves can be reflectively enhanced, and frequent bathing can enhance the adaptability to cold stress and has health care effects such as heath strengthening and disease prevention.

水温在 34~37℃时,对大脑皮质有抑制作用,可以降低神经系统的兴奋性,有明显的镇静作用,对头痛、失眠、神经官能症及脑血管后遗症等有一定疗效。

With water temperature of 34-37℃, the cerebral cortex can be inhibited, the excitability of neural systems can be reduced with significant tranquilizing, with a certain therapeutic effect to headache, insomnia, neurosis, and sequela of cerebrovascular diseases.

（二）水的浮力作用

（Ⅱ）Water Buoyancy

温泉的矿物质含量越高，比重就越大，浸浴时产生的浮力也越大，人体浸浴时所感受到的实际重量明显减少。

The more mineral content the hot spring contains, the higher specific gravity it has; the more buoyancy the hot spring generates during the immersion bath, the less actual weight the body feels.

由于体重"变轻"，人的运动变得比较容易，故对某些肌肉、关节及神经系统疾病所致的肢体运动障碍的康复有利。

Due to decrease of the body weight, the movement of human body becomes easier, which is beneficial to the recovery of limb movement disturbance caused by certain muscular, joint and neural system diseases.

（三）水的压力作用

（Ⅲ）Water Pressure

人在温泉中，全身要承受水的压力，会感觉呼气易、吸气难，这可以锻炼机体的呼吸功能，加强机体代谢。

In the hot spring, due to the fact that the whole body is under water pressure, it is easy to inhale but difficult to exhale, which can strengthen the respiratory function of the body and enhance the metabolism of the body.

此外，这种压力会压迫体表的血管和淋巴管，促使血液向心回流，由此引起体液的再分配。

In addition, this pressure can constrict the blood vessels and lymphatic vessels of the body surface, which causes blood to flow back to the heart, thus resulting in redistribution of body fluids.

如果在浴池里人为地使水流加速，例如制造波浪等，则会发挥温泉浴的机械刺激作用，这样可加速血液和淋巴液的循环。

If water flow is artificially accelerated, for example, by making waves in the bathing pool, then mechanical stimulation of the hot spring bath can be provided, which can accelerate the circulation of blood and lymph fluid.

（四）化学刺激作用

（Ⅳ）Chemical Stimulus

这是矿泉浴的特异性治疗作用。

This is the specific therapeutic effect of hot spring bath.

在浸浴过程中,有些矿物质成分可通过皮肤进入体内,有的虽不能经皮肤吸收,但却能附着于皮肤对神经末梢产生作用。

In the process of immersion bath, some mineral compositions can penetrate into the body through skin while some can be effective to nerve terminals by attaching to skin even though they cannot be absorbed through skin.

还有一些气体成分则通过呼吸道进入体内而发挥作用。

In addition, some gas compositions come into play by entering the body through respiratory tract.

二、常见温泉种类及适应证

Ⅱ. Common Types and Indications of Hot Springs

不同的温泉有不同的治疗作用,所以人们按照温泉水所含化学成分和水温高低进行了分类。

Therapeutic effects vary with different hot springs, therefore hot spring water is classified according to the included chemical compositions and water temperature.

（一）单纯泉

（Ⅰ）Simple spring

水温在 25℃以上,可溶性固体成分含量在每升 1 000mg 以下。

It is above 25℃ and its soluble solid composition content is below 1 000mg per litre.

主要靠产热产生治疗作用,温水有镇痛和加快新陈代谢,促进血液循环,通经活络等作用。

It produces therapeutic effects mainly by generating heat and warm water can ease pain, accelerate metabolism, promote blood circulation, dredge meridians and activate collaterals.

温浴可治疗风湿性关节炎、类风湿关节炎、慢性支气管炎、慢性咽炎、便秘、神经性皮炎等皮肤病。

Warm spring bath can be used to treat rheumatic arthritis, rheumatoid arthritis, chronic bronchitis, chronic pharyngitis, constipation, neurodermatitis and other dermatoses.

(二) 重碳酸土类泉
(Ⅱ) Bicarbonate soil type spring

水中含有可溶性固体成分的总量在每升 1 000mg 以上。

Its soluble solid composition content is above 1 000mg per litre in total.

其主要成分中阴离子是重碳酸根离子,阳离子是钙、镁离子。

In its major compositions, the anions are bicarbonate ions, and the cations are calcium and magnesium ions.

钙离子除对皮肤黏膜炎症有效外,还有兴奋神经、降低血管内皮细胞通透性作用。

Calcium ions are not only effective in treating skin mucosal inflammation, but also in exciting nerves and reducing vascular endothelial cell permeability.

温浴可治疗心瓣膜病、心肌衰弱、肺气肿、变应性鼻炎等。

Warm spring bath can be used to treat valvular disease, amyocardia, pulmonary emphysema, allergic rhinitis, etc.

(三) 重碳酸钠泉
(Ⅲ) Sodium bicarbonate spring

水中含可溶性固体成分每升 1 000mg 以上,以阴离子重碳酸根离子、阳离子钠离子为主要成分,泉水有类似肥皂的作用,可使皮肤乳化,使皮肤显得光滑。

Its soluble solid composition content is above 1 000mg per litre, which mainly includes bicarbonate ions as anions and sodium ions as cations, and the spring has the function of soap to emulsify and smooth skin.

温浴可治疗前列腺炎、不孕症、风湿病、腰肌劳损、神经性皮炎、皮肤疹痒、各种皮肤癣症。

This kind of warm bath can be used to treat prostatitis, infertility, rheumatoid, lumbar muscle strain, neurodermatitis, cutaneous prurigo, cutaneous tinea, etc.

（四）食盐泉

（Ⅳ）Common salt spring

是指温泉中含盐量在每升 1 000mg 以上的泉水，主要成分为氯离子和钠离子，浴后温暖感很强，并能刺激皮肤，使皮肤血管扩张，增进体表血液循环，加速汗腺和皮脂腺的分泌，加快胃肠蠕动，对神经性疼痛、风湿病和妇女冷感症、肥胖症均有疗效。

It refers to the spring with the salt content of over 1 000mg per litre, mainly including chloride ions and sodium ions, which provides very strong warmth after bathing and stimulate skin for dermal vasodilatation, improvement of blood circulation of the body surface, acceleration of the secretion of the sweat gland, and sebaceous gland and acceleration of gastrointestinal peristalsis, having therapeutic effects on neuropathic pain, rheumatism, women's sense of coldness and obesity.

（五）铁泉

（Ⅴ）Iron spring

温泉中含有二价或三价铁离子每升 10mg 以上，铁多以离子形式存在，可治疗慢性风湿病、腰腿痛、痔疮、月经不调、各种皮肤癣症等。

It contains over 10mg of ferrous or ferric ion per litre, with iron mostly existing in the form of ion, which can be used to treat chronic rheumatism, pain in waist and lower extremities, hemorrhoids, irregular menstruation, skin tinea, etc.

（六）硫黄泉

（Ⅵ）Sulfur spring

水中主要含游离硫化氢，硫黄总量在每升 1mg 以上，能溶解角质，软化皮肤，并有消炎杀菌、通经活络、祛寒止痛的作用，温浴可治疗糖尿病、风湿痛、腰腿疼、风湿性关节炎、皮肤瘙痒、癣疥疮疖等。

It mainly contains free hydrogen sulphide, with the total sulphur content of over 1mg per litre. It dissolves cutin, softens the skin and has the function of anti-inflammation, disinfection, dredging meridians, activating collaterals, dispelling cold and relieving pain. This kind of warm bath can be used to treat diabetes, rheumatism, lumbago and leg pain, rheumatic arthritis , cutaneous pruritus, tinea, scabies, sores, furuncles, etc.

（七）放射能泉

（Ⅶ）Radioactive spring

水中含镭每升 10^{-7}mg 以上，氡在 30×10^{-10}Ci 以上时称为放射能泉。

It contains over 10^{-7}mg of radium per litre and over 30×10^{-10} Ci of radon.

放射能泉一般都有刺激作用，特别对细胞分裂旺盛的组织易起控制作用。

The radioactive spring is generally stimulative, particularly has the function of easily controlling the tissues where cell division is active.

当人体浴用这种含适量氡的温泉水时，氡的电离辐射作用能够调节和改善神经系统，平衡中枢神经系统的兴奋和抑制功能，促进睡眠，减轻疼痛，并使血压下降。

When the hot spring water with a moderate amount of radon is used for bathing, the ionizing radiation of radon can adjust and improve the neural system, and balance the excitation and inhibition of central neural system, so as to promote sleep, alleviate pain and reduce blood pressure.

可用来防治癌症、贫血、支气管哮喘、白细胞减少症、心肌衰弱、神经衰弱、偏瘫等。

It can be used to prevent and treat cancers, anemia, bronchial asthma, leucopenia, amyocardia, neurasthenia, hemiplegia, etc.

特别是对糖尿病患者可减少血糖和尿糖，具有良好的医疗作用。

It has a good medical effect particularly in reducing blood sugar and urine sugar of the diabetic.

人们在进行温泉疗法时，首先应该经过医生的全面检查并在医生的指导下，根据每处温泉所含的不同成分和每种疾病的特性，进行针对性选择。

For the warm bath treatment, the overall checkup for the acceptor should be first given by the doctor, and under the direction of the doctor, according to the different compositions contained in each hot spring and the characteristics of each disease, the pertinent selection is performed.

做到因人而异,对症"下水"。

Hot springs vary from person to person for different treatments.

三、温泉浴的临床适应证与禁忌证

Ⅲ. Clinical Indications and Contraindications of Hot Spring Bath

（一）适应证

（Ⅰ）Indications

1. 亚健康状态　温泉浴适用于许多亚健康状态,如对失眠、抑郁、神经衰弱、精力不足、长期乏力等具有优良的改善效果。

1. Sub-health states　The hot spring bath is suitable to many sub-health states such as insomnia,depression,neurasthenia,aneuria,long-term exhaustion, etc.

2. 美容与皮肤病　温泉浴美容,是借洗浴时温泉浴热水对肌肤的刺激作用和温泉浴水中富含的硫化氢、氟、偏硼酸等多种有益人体健康的矿物质和微量元素的"药浴"作用,使腠理疏通、气血流畅,从而达到养颜目的。

2. Beauty treatment and dermatosis　The warm spring bath for beauty treatment can dredge the striae of skin and the texture of the subcutaneous flesh and promote qi and blood flow for skin beautification through the stimulation of skin by the hot spring water and through the medical actions of multiple beneficial minerals and trace elements contained in hot spring water such as hydrogen sulphide,fluorine,metaboric acid,etc.

温泉浴对于许多慢性皮肤病也有着良好的辅助治疗效果,如银屑病、神经性皮炎、皮肤瘙痒、痤疮、癣疥疮疖、皮肤疹痒、鸡眼等。

The hot spring bath is also effective in the adjuvant treatment of many chronic dermatoses such as psoriasis,neurodermatitis,cutaneous pruritus,acnes, tinea,scabies,sores,furuncles,cutaneous prurigo,helosis,etc.

3. 风湿骨病康复治疗　风湿性关节炎、类风湿关节炎、腰肌劳损、腰腿疼、关节僵硬、肢体麻痹、颈腰症候群、肌肉酸痛、肌腱炎、神经炎、偏瘫、截瘫等。

3. Rehabilitation of rheumatoid bone diseases　Rheumatic arthritis, rheumatoid arthritis,lumbar muscle strain,lumbago and leg pain,anchylosis,limb paralysis, cervico-lumbar syndrome, muscular soreness, myotenositis, neuritis, hemiplegia, paraplegia, etc.

4. 其他慢性病　除上述疾病外,温泉浴疗法还对许多其他慢性病有着很好的疗效,如痔疮、疮口收敛愈合、慢性支气管炎、慢性咽炎、便秘、变应性鼻炎、前列腺炎、肥胖症、糖尿病、贫血等。

4. Other chronic diseases　In addition to the above diseases, the hot spring bath treatment is also effective to many other chronic diseases such as hemorrhoid, wound healing, chronic bronchitis, chronic pharyngitis, constipation, allergic rhinitis, prostatitis, obesity, diabetes, anemia, etc.

(二) 禁忌证

(Ⅱ) Contraindications

温泉浴不是"包治百病",有以下情况者请不要进行浴疗:一切患有急性发热性疾病、急性传染病、病情恶化的慢性及并发的化脓过程。

Hot spring bath is not guaranteed to cure all diseases, and bath treatment is not allowed for the following: all of acute febrile diseases, acute infectious diseases, and chronic and complicated pyogenic process caused by exacerbation.

一切器官的结核性疾病:如肺结核、骨结核、生殖器官结核、肾结核、淋巴结核等。

All of tuberculous diseases in organs: such as pulmonary tuberculosis, bone tuberculosis, genital tuberculosis, renal tuberculosis and lymphatic tuberculosis.

病情加重的恶性贫血、晚期原发性红细胞增多症、白血病等。

Aggravated pernicious anemia, advanced primary erythrocytosis, leukemia, etc.

任何原因引起的恶病质、恶性肿瘤。

Cachexia and malignant neoplasm from any causes.

出血性及有出血倾向的疾病。

Hemorrhagic diseases and diseases with hemorrhagic tendency.

代偿不全的心脏病伴有血管硬化的高血压、动脉硬化症。

Decompensated heart disease with angiosclerotic hypertension and atherosclerosis.

各种原因引起的精神病。

Psychoses from various causes.

有慢性阑尾炎史的适应证患者。

And eligible patients who suffered from chronic appendicitis.

大脑及脊髓实质性病变：如帕金森病和侧索硬化、后索变性及侧索后索联合变性。

Solid lesions of cerebrum and spinal cord：such as Parkinson disease and lateral sclerosis，posterior funiculus degeneration and combined degeneration of lateral funiculus and posterior funiculus.

一切急性期与有传染性的性病（梅毒、淋病患者）。

All of acute-phase diseases and infectious venereal diseases（syphilis and gonorrhoea patients）.

酒醉、饱食（1小时内）及空腹（饭前30分钟）后，不宜入浴。

It is not suitable for persons who are drunken or full（within 1 hour），or whose stomach is empty（30 minutes before a meal）.

前两者会因为流经胃部的血液减少而致消化不良，甚至休克；空腹则容易疲劳。

The former two conditions can lead to dyspepsia and even shock due to the reduction of the blood flowing through the stomach；an empty stomach easily leads to fatigue.

女性生理期前后，怀孕初期或后期的孕妇。

Women before and after menstruation，and pregnant women during early and late stages of pregnancy.

（三）温泉浴治疗的注意事项

（Ⅲ）Cautions for Hot Spring Bath Treatment

1. **温泉浴不当会患上皮肤病**　例如青磺泉（是地下水中渗入火山气体，经酸化后混入少量地表水而成，其特征是温度高可达沸点且酸性强），pH值在1~2之间，属于强酸范围。

1. **Improper hot spring bath will cause dermatosis**　For example，Qinghuang hot spring（It is formed by the underground water infiltrated with volcanic gas

and mixed with a small amount of surface water after acidification, and its feature lies in the temperature as high as the boiling point and its strong acidity) has pH between 1 and 2, which falls within the scope of strong acid.

泡在酸性比较强的温泉里,那些本身皮肤比较干燥或患湿疹、特应性皮炎等问题的人得温泉皮肤病的可能性很大。

People themselves with dry skin or such diseases as eczema and atopic dermatitis are more likely to suffer from dermatosis if they take baths in strong acidic acidic hot spring.

2. 温泉性氟中毒 因温泉普遍含有较高的氟,会引起周围居民罹患地方性氟中毒,称为温泉性氟中毒。

2. Hot spring fluorine poisoning The hot spring generally contains high-level fluorine and this will cause the surrounding residents to suffer from endemic fluorine poisoning, which is therefore referred to as hot spring fluorine poisoning.

高氟温泉不仅可以引起氟斑牙,也可造成氟骨症。

The hot spring with high-level fluorine will not only cause dental fluorosis but also cause skeletal fluorosis.

氟骨症的检出率与温泉的含氟量呈近似正相关。

There is an approximate positive correlation between the detection rate of skeletal fluorosis and the fluorine content of hot spring.

3. 温泉浴室内氡放射对人体的危害 长期大量吸入氡及其子体会对健康产生危害。

3. Damage of radon emission in the hot spring to human body Inhaling too much radon and its progenies for a long time will be harmful to people's health.

氡在浴疗时不断地从池水中逸散于空气中,使浴室内及周围空气中的氡及子体的放射性比活度明显增高。

During the bath therapy, radon can constantly escape from the pool water into the air, which significantly increases the specific radioactivity of radon and its progenies in the bathroom and the surrounding air.

4. 温泉浴池水细菌污染 温泉浴池水有利于细菌的滋生繁殖,成为接触传染和介水传染病传播的重大隐患。

4. Bacterial contamination of water in the hot spring bathing pool　Hot spring water is conducive to breeding of bacteria, which is the severe potential danger of contact transmission and water-borne infection disease transmission.

参 考 文 献
References

［1］蒲昭和.温泉浴为何有保健功效[J].老年人,2008(2):57-57.

［2］王邵林,姚强,徐丽,等.矿泉对人体生理作用机制的探讨[J].中国疗养医学,2004(2):13-14.

［3］郭世先,葛本伟,陈辉,等.温泉与健康[J].国外医学(医学地理分册),2005,26(2):90-93.

［4］李日邦.中国的温泉及温泉型氟中毒的地理分布[J].中国地方病学杂志,1995(2):119-120.

［5］马吉英.室内氡对人体健康的危害及防护[J].中国辐射卫生,2012,21(4):506-508.

第四章　熥　疗　法
Chapter 4　Tong Therapy

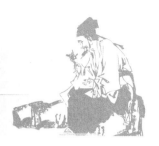

第一节　中药熥疗法
Section 1　Tong Therapy of TCM

一、疗法简介

I. Therapy Profile

中药熥疗,又叫熨疗,其历史悠久,源远流长,最早的文字记载见于《素问·调经论》:"病在骨,淬针药熨。"《素问·血气形志》:"形苦志乐,病生于筋,治之以熨引。"《史记·扁鹊仓公列传》中记述了秦越人用熨法治疗虢太子的尸厥病,司马贞《索隐》中提到:"毒熨,谓毒病之处,以药物熨帖。"《圣济经》记载:"熨,资火气以舒寒结,凡筋肉挛急,顽痹不仁,熨能通之也……"

Tong therapy of TCM, also called as a hot medicinal compress therapy, has a long history. The earliest written records on it are found in the *Plain Questions-Theory of Regulating Meridians*, which records that "for the bone diseases, heated needle and hot medicinal compress therapy of Chinese Traditional Medicine are applied." The *Plain Questions-Theory about Blood-Qi-Body-Mind* records that "Once the patients have excessive physical labor and leisurely mood, tendon and ligament may have a disease, so the hot medicinal compress therapy is applied." The *Records of the Grand Historian-Collected Biographies of Bian Que and Cang Gong* records that Qin yueren treated cadaverous syncope disease of prince of the Guo state by hot medicinal compress therapy. Si Mazhen's *Suo Yin* mentions that "toxin hot medicinal compress means that the medicine hot medicinal compress is applied at the toxin positions." The *Classic of Holy*

Benevolence records that "hot medicinal compress uses heat to dispel cold-stagnation, so for muscular contracture and tender spasm, and intractable blockage with numbness, the hot medicinal compress can be applied to effect a cure…"

清代关于熨疗法已有较详尽的论述。

The hot medicinal compress therapy had been discussed in detail at the Qing dynasty.

中药熥疗法,是在古代熨法的基础之上,结合现代人体质和疾病进行的改良。

The Tong therapy of TCM is an improved hot medicinal compress therapy based on the ancient hot medicinal compress therapy and combining with the physical constitution and diseases of modern people.

中药熥疗是将装有多味中药的药袋放入蒸锅内蒸熥加热,然后置于体表特定部位进行持续加温的一种中药外治疗法。

The Tong therapy of TCM is an external therapy of TCM which puts the medicine packages containing several kinds of CMMs into a boiler to steam and heat and then puts the medicine packages on the specific positions of the body surface to continuously heat up.

其通过皮肤直接给药,热效应持久,药力和热力联合作用于肌表,内传经络脏腑起到治病调理的作用(见图 4-1)。

The medicine is directly administered through the skin. The heat effect is lasting. The medicine efficacy and the heating power act together onto the body surface, then the actions further spread to the meridians, collaterals and zang-fu organs, so as to effect the function of treating diseases and regulating the body (see Fig. 4-1).

中药熥疗能使腠理疏松、气血流畅,具有祛风散寒、止痛消炎、温经通络、利水消肿等作用。

The Tong therapy of TCM can make the striae loose, and flow of qi-blood smooth, with the functions of expelling wind and removing cold, relieving pain and eliminating inflammation, warming meridians and dredging collaterals, inducing urination to alleviate edema, etc.

在临床上具有操作简便、安全无痛、经济有效的优势,受到广大患者的一致好评。

The Tong therapy of TCM is clinically easy to operate, safe, painless, economical and effective. So it is highly praised by most patients.

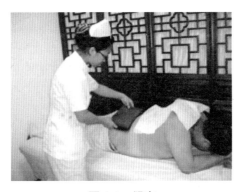

图 4-1　熥疗
Fig. 4-1　Tong therapy

二、操作规范

Ⅱ. Operation Specifications

(一) 操作前准备

(Ⅰ) Preparation before Operation

1. 器械准备　双层蒸锅、电磁炉、持物钳、一次性手套、无菌布、棉被等。

1. Instrument preparation　Double boiler, induction cooker, holding forceps, disposable gloves, sterile cloth, cotton quilt, etc.

2. 患者准备　根据穴位依次选取相应的体位进行治疗。

2. Preparation for patient　The corresponding body positions of the patient are selected in proper sequence according to acupoints.

3. 皮肤评估　包括色泽、弹性,有无水肿、出血、蜘蛛痣、肝掌、异常隆起、包块及皮下脂肪层厚度等方面指标。

3. Skin assessment　Such indicators as color, elasticity, whether there are conditions of edema, bleeding, spider nevus, liver palm, anomalous prominence, lump and fat lining thickness should be assessed.

（二）详细操作步骤

（Ⅱ）Detailed Operation Procedures

1. 根据病情选择适当的方剂,将研磨成粉剂并调配好的中草药置于布袋内(实际药包大小和重量可按操作者需求和患者治疗部位进行调整)。

1. According to the patient's conditions, an appropriate prescription is selected and is ground into powder, and the dispensed Chinese herbal medicine is put into the cloth bag (the actual size and weight of the medicine package can be adjusted according to the operators' requirements and the patients' positions treated).

首次使用蒸3~4小时,此后每次使用约待水开再蒸熨30分钟即可(见图4-2)。

For the first use, the cloth bag is steamed for about 3-4 hours, and then is steamed for about 30 minutes after water boiling every time before use (see Fig. 4-2).

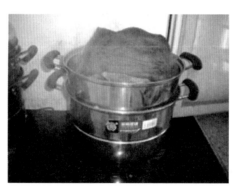

图 4-2　加热用具
Fig. 4-2　Heating appliance

2. 根据患者疾病的不同部位选取仰卧、俯卧、侧卧位或坐位进行治疗。

2. According to the different positions of the patients' diseases, the supine position, prone position, lateral position or sitting position are selected to conduct treatment.

患者就位后,检查治疗部位有无皮肤破损、红肿或感觉障碍。

After the patients are in position, the treated positions are inspected to ensure whether there are damage, redness or sensory disorder of the skin.

无碍后使用清洁湿毛巾擦拭治疗部位。

The clean moist towels are used to wipe down the treated positions after there is no problem.

3. 待药包彻底蒸透,施术者戴好一次性手套,用持物钳夹出一个煹疗药包,晾至 40~50℃,再从锅里取出另外一个蒸煹加热好的药包,晾至 60~70℃。

3. After the medicine packages are thoroughly steamed, the operator wears disposable gloves, clips a medicine package of the Tong therapy with forceps and cools it to 40-50℃, and then takes out another steamed and heated medicine package from a boiler and cools it to 60-70℃.

将后取出的温度高的药包放在先前取出的药包上面,同时把两个药包拿起,将温度低的药包平整放置于患者的治疗部位上,随后在药包上加盖无菌布,最后覆以薄棉被保温。

The operator puts the latter medicine package with high temperature on the former medicine package, takes up both medicine packages, puts them onto the treated positions of the patients, and then covers up with sterile cloth, and finally covers up with a thin cotton quilt to preserve heat.

10~15 分钟后两药包位置互换以保证治疗温度(见图 4-3)。

After 10-15 minutes, the positions of two medicine packages are exchanged to ensure the temperature of treatment(see Fig. 4-3).

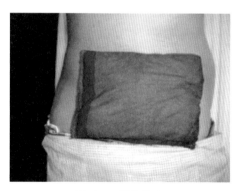

图 4-3　背部治疗
Fig. 4-3　Back treatment

4. 治疗结束后施术者将药包收起,使用卫生纸将患者治疗部位擦拭干净,待患者汗出停止后方可离开。

4. After the treatment, the operator packs the medicine packages up, and uses the tissues to clean the treated positions of the patients. The operator cannot leave until the patient stops sweating.

(三) 治疗时间及疗程
(Ⅲ) Treatment Time and Course

每次治疗时间为 20~30 分钟, 15 天为 1 个疗程, 2 个疗程之间间隔 4~5 天。

The treatment time lasts 20-30 minutes every time, a period of 15 days constitutes one course and the interval between two courses is 4-5 days.

(四) 注意事项
(Ⅳ) Precautions

1. **施术者注意** 药包使用前需要保持干燥, 治疗期间施术者于床旁停留 1 分钟, 观察患者对药包的耐热程度, 观察患者治疗部位是否有红肿热痛、是否起水疱等。

1. **Precautions for operator** The medicine package needs to keep dry before use. The operator stays for one minute at the side of the bed during the treatment to observe the degree of heat resistance of the patient to the medicine package, and observe whether there are redness, swelling, heat and pain at the treated positions of the patients and whether there are blisters, etc.

患者治疗部位皮肤近期如使用过外用药膏, 可能提高皮肤敏感性, 注意烫伤及不良反应的发生。

If ointment has been applied to the skin of the treated position of the patient in the near future, the skin sensitivity can be increased, so the attention to occurrence of scalds and adverse reactions should be paid.

敏感皮肤患者, 治疗时间应适当缩短。

For the patients with sensitive skin, the treatment time should be appropriately shortened.

2. **嘱患者注意** 勿空腹或过饱进行本项治疗, 治疗前后应适当补充温开水。

2. **The patient should be asked to pay attention to the following** Do not keep the stomach empty or overeaten during this treatment; drink warm water

appropriately before and after this treatment.

治疗后出现皮肤表面发红、汗出属正常现象,但应注意避风寒。

The skin surface may turn red and perspire after treatment, which is a normal phenomenon, but the patient should pay attention to keep away from wind and cold.

勿用化妆品,勿洗澡。

Do not apply cosmetics, do not have a bath.

尤其注意头颈部、腰部四肢、足部的保暖,治疗后待汗止后方可离开。

Particularly keep the head, neck, waist, arms, legs and feet warm; and do not leave the treatment room after the treatment until sweating stops.

皮肤可能出现局部泛红、肿胀,甚至脱屑及色素沉着等反应。

There may be redness, swelling and even desquamation, pigmentation and other reactions in local skin.

这种情况多为中药熥疗的疗效体现,数日后可自然消失。

This condition mostly reflects the curative effect of the Tong therapy of TCM and can be disappeared naturally days later.

三、临床应用

Ⅲ. Clinical Application

(一) 适应证
(Ⅰ) Indications

由寒邪侵袭所致的一些骨科、软伤科和内科疾病。

Some orthopedic diseases, soft tissue injury diseases and internal diseases caused by invasion of pathogenic cold to the body.

如颈腰椎疾病,风湿性关节炎、类风湿关节炎,退行性骨关节炎,劳损性骨病,骨质增生等骨关节疾病;

Osteoarticular diseases such as cervical and lumbar spine disease, rheumatic arthritis, rheumatoid arthritis, degenerative osteoarthritis, strain osteopathy and hyperosteogeny;

肌肉劳损,扭伤、挫伤后所致的肌肉疼痛等;

muscle strain, muscular pain caused by sprain and contusion, etc.;

以及胃痛、便秘、泄泻、慢性前列腺炎等疾病。

and stomach ache, constipation, diarrhea, chronic prostatitis, etc.

中药熥疗热效应及药物效应叠加,热效应尤为突出,因其较热,适合身体比较强壮的患者。

The heat effect and drug effect of the Tong therapy of TCM are multiplied. The heat effect is particularly prominent. Because it is hotter, the therapy is suitable for the patients with stronger constitution.

（二）处方示例

（Ⅱ）Prescription Examples

1. 膝关节炎、颈椎病、腰椎间盘突出症（风寒湿型及气滞血瘀型）

1. Gonitis, cervical spondylosis and prolapse of lumbar intervertebral disc (types of wind-cold-dampness and qi-stagnation and blood stasis)

（1）临床表现:患处重着疼痛,肌肉酸痛,关节屈伸不利,得热痛减,舌苔薄白,脉浮弦或沉紧。

(1) Clinical manifestation: Heavy pain in the affected area, aches and pain of muscles, inconvenient flexion and extension of joints, pain relieved by heat, thin white coating of tongue, stringy floating pulse or deep pulse.

（2）配方:白芥子 20g、甘遂 15g、延胡索 15g、大黄 20g、芒硝 20g、伸筋草 10g、透骨草 10g、乳香 10g、没药 10g。

(2) Prescription: White mustard seed (20g), gansui root (15g), yanhusuo (15g), rhubarb root and rhizome (20g), mirabilite (20g), common clubmoss herb (10g), speranskia herb (10g), frankincense (10g), and myrrh (10g).

（3）膝关节取穴:内外膝眼穴、血海、梁丘。

(3) Acupoint selection of knee joint: Internal and external Xiyan, Xuehai and Liangqiu.

颈椎取穴:大椎、夹脊。

Acupoint selection of cervical vertebra: Dazhui and Jiaji.

腰部取穴:肾俞、委中、腰阳关、命门。

Acupoint selection of waist:Shenshu, Weizhong, Yaoyangguan and Mingmen.

2. 胃痛(脾胃虚寒型)

2. Stomachache(type of deficiency–cold in spleen and stomach)

(1) 临床表现:胃痛隐隐,绵绵不休,喜温喜按,空腹痛甚,得食则缓,舌淡苔白,脉虚弱或迟缓。

(1) Clinical manifestation:Persistent dull stomachache with a preference of warmth and pressing,pain aggravated as stomach being empty and relieved by food intake,pale tongue with whitish coating,and weak or slow pulse.

(2) 配方:小茴香 20g、木香 10g、乌药 20g、肉桂 10g、艾叶 20g、白芷 10g、白芥子 10g、胡椒 10g、生姜 20g、大枣 10g。

(2) Prescription:Fennel(20g),common aucklandia root(10g),combined spicebush root(20g),cassia bark(10g),argy wormwood leaves(20g),dahurian angelica root(10g),white mustard seed(10g),pepper(10g),fresh ginger(20g),and Chinese date(10g).

(3) 取穴:中脘、气海、神阙。

(3) Acupoint selection:Zhongwan,Qihai and Shenque.

3. 泄泻(脾胃虚弱型)

3. Diarrhea(type of spleen and stomach deficiency type)

(1) 临床表现:大便时泄时溏,食少,食后脘闷不舒,面色萎黄,舌质淡,苔白,脉细弱。

(1) Clinical manifestations:Diarrhea or loose stool,poor appetite,epigastric stuffiness after meal,sallow complexion,pale tongue with white coating,and thready and weak pulse.

(2) 配方:丁香 20g、肉桂 10g、艾叶 20g、雄黄 10g、冰片 5g、干姜 20g、细辛 10g、川椒 10g、白胡椒 10g、吴茱萸 10g、炮姜 20g。

(2) Prescription:Clove(20g),cassia bark(10g),argy wormwood leaves (20g),realgar(10g),borneol(5g),dried ginger(20g),manchurian wildginger (10g),Sichuan pepper(10g),white pepper(10g),medicinal evodia fruit(10g)and

baked ginger(20g).

（3）取穴：神阙、天枢、气海、关元、足三里。

（3）Acupoint selection：Shenque，Tianshu，Qihai，Guanyuan and Zusanli.

4. 前列腺炎（肾阳不足型）

4. Prostatitis（insufficiency of kidney-yang type）

（1）临床表现：小腹胀满，时欲小便不得出，或量少无力，面色㿠白，畏寒肢冷，舌淡胖，苔薄白，脉沉细或弱。

（1）Clinical manifestations：Lower abdominal distension，frequent urination with difficulty to urinate，or oliguria or acraturesis，pale complexion，intolerance to cold and cold limbs，pale and enlarged tongue with white and thin coating，and deep thready or weak pulse.

（2）配方：葱白 20g、芒硝 10g、明矾 20g、白胡椒 10g、吴茱萸 15g、大黄 20g、王不留行 15g、花椒 10g、牛膝 15g、冰片 5g。

（2）Prescription：Onion stalk(20g)，mirabilite(10g)，alum(20g)，white pepper(10g)，medicinal evodia fruit(15g)，rhubarb root and rhizome(20g)，cowherb seed(15g)，pricklyash peel(10g)，twotoothed achyranthes root(15g) and borneol(5g).

（3）取穴：中极、关元。

（3）Acupoint selection：Zhongji and Guanyuan.

5. 便秘（脾肾阳虚型）

5. Constipation（type of yang deficiency of spleen and kidney）

（1）临床表现：大便干或不干，排出困难，小便清长，面色㿠白，腹中冷痛，舌淡苔白，脉沉迟。

（1）Clinical manifestation：Dry or wet stool with difficulty to defecate，copious and clear urine，pale complexion，cold pain in abdomen，pale tongue with whitish coating，slow and deep pulse.

（2）配方：大黄 30g、甘遂 15g、芒硝 20g、葱白 15g、丁香 10g、大蒜 20g、生姜 10g、薄荷 15g。

（2）Prescription：Rhubarb root and rhizome(30g)，gansui root(15g)， mirabilite(20g),onion stalk(15g),clove(10g),garlic(20g),fresh ginger(10g),and peppermint(15g).

（3）取穴：支沟、天枢、大横。

（3）Acupoint selection：Zhigou，Tianshu and Daheng.

（三）禁忌证
（Ⅲ）Contraindications

1. **内科疾病**　体质虚弱,高热,结核,恶性肿瘤,出血倾向,重症糖尿病,甲状腺功能亢进,心脏病,高血压,肾功能不全,感染性皮肤病,温热感觉障碍,重症循环衰竭等疾病。

1. **Internal Diseases**　The Tong therapy of TCM is contraindicated for the patients who have diseases such as constitutional weakness,hyperpyrexia, tuberculosis,malignant tumor,hemorrhagic tendency,severe diabetes, hyperthyroidism,heart disease,hypertension,renal insufficiency,infectious skin diseases,warm sensation disorder and severe circulatory failure.

2. **妇科禁忌**　孕妇腹部、腰骶部及某些可促进子宫收缩的穴位,如合谷、三阴交等应禁止中药熥疗,有些药物如麝香等孕妇禁用,以免引起流产。

2. **Contraindication for gynecology**　The Tong therapy of TCM should be prohibited from application for pregnant women at the abdomen,lumbosacral portion and some acupoints such as Hegu and Sanyinjiao,which may cause uterine contraction. For pregnant women,some medicines such as musk are also prohibited to avoid abortion.

经期禁用。

It is prohibited during menstrual period.

3. **其他**　局部皮肤有创伤、溃疡、感染或有严重的皮肤病者禁用。

3. **Other conditions**　The Tong therapy of TCM is contraindicated for patients whose local skins have wound,ulcer and infection or who have severe skin diseases.

对药物成分过敏者禁用,6岁以下儿童禁用。

It is prohibited for the patients who are allergic to drug ingredients and for the children under the age of six.

（四）不良反应及处理方法

（Ⅳ）Adverse Reactions and Treatment

1. **烫伤处理** 烫伤出现较小的水疱可待其自行吸收，若水疱较大则应用无菌针头吸出水疱中的组织液并涂以烫伤药膏以避免感染，并促进伤口愈合。

1. Treatment for scalds   The smaller blisters of scalds can be naturally absorbed. For the larger blisters, the sterile needles should be used to suction out the tissue fluids, and then the scald ointment is applied to avoid infection and promote wound healing.

2. **过敏反应处理** 及时停药，蒸馏水清洗局部，如有其他系统反应，应及时转诊。

2. Treatment for Allergy   Immediately stop medication and clean the local skin with distilled water. If there are other systematic responses, the referral should be done timely for treatment.

3. **其他不良反应处理** 由于药包较热，有可能出现心悸、心慌、血压升高等症状，嘱患者静卧监测血压，如未缓解再对症治疗。

3. Treatment for other adverse reactions   As the medicine package is hotter, it is possible to produce the symptoms of palpitation and elevation of blood pressure, etc. Such being the case, the patients should be asked to lie quietly for monitoring the blood pressure. If the symptoms persist, specific treatment should be performed accordingly.

参 考 文 献

References

［1］王野,白一辰. 熥疗结合推拿治疗梨状肌损伤综合征 43 例临床观察［J］. 辽宁中医杂志,2015,42（9）:1743-1745.

［2］张杰,胡海,李志刚,等. 推拿手法配合中药熥疗治疗腰背肌筋膜炎 60 例临床疗效分析［J］. 中国中医药科技,2017,24（1）:81-82.

［3］张慧玲. 中药熥疗治疗原发性痛经 136 例［J］. 陕西中医,2008（3）:268-269.

［4］杨百京,陈风琴. 中药熥疗治疗腰痛 86 例观察［J］. 新疆中医药,2003（2）:22-23.

第二节 中药热罨包疗法
Section 2 Therapy of TCM Hot Package

一、疗法简介
I. Therapy Profile

中药热罨包治疗是用浸满中药药液的滤纸置于身体的患病部位或特定穴位上(如图 4-4),通过放置热罨包使局部的毛细血管扩张,血液循环加速,使滤纸上的中药渗透到患处穴位,利用其温热之力达到温经通络、调和气血、祛湿散寒的作用。

Therapy of TCM hot package is to place the filter paper soaked with CMM liquid on the diseased area or specific acupoints (see Fig. 4-4), by the action of hot package to dilate the local capillaries and promote blood circulation, so as to make the CMM on the filter paper penetrate into the acupoints of the affected areas and thus through use its warm power to achieve the functions of warming meridians and dredging collaterals, harmonizing qi and blood, and dispelling cold and removing dampness.

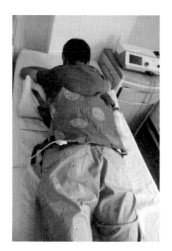

图 4-4 热罨包
Fig. 4-4 Hot package

此种治疗方法是从中药热敷即"熨法"改革而来,不但发挥了其热效应,还能使治疗温度更加容易掌控,与中药熻疗和中药熏药治疗比起来,出现烫伤等不良反应的概率大大降低,适应范围更广,使用起来更安全,尤其适用于身材瘦弱、体弱久病、老年人及儿童等。

This therapy is reformed from the TCM hot compress, i.e. "hot medicinal compress". It not only exerts its thermal effect but also makes the treatment temperature easier to control. Compared with Tong therapy and Fumigation therapy of TCM, this therapy has small probabilities of scald and other adverse reactions. So it has wider range of application and it is safe to use, being especially suitable for the persons with a weak constitution, or patients with chronic diseases, or the elderly, or children.

二、操作技术

Ⅱ. Operation Techniques

(一) 操作前准备

(Ⅰ) Preparation before Operation

1. **材料准备**　以中医基础理论为指导,辨证论治,按照一定的剂量煎制药物,将煎好的药汤趁热倒入不锈钢盘内,根据患者的治疗部位裁取滤纸尺寸后将滤纸浸入药汤(如图 4-5)。

1. **Material preparation**　Guided by basic theory of TCM, the doctor should give treatment based on syndrome differentiation, decoct and process medicines in a certain dose, pour the decocted medical liquid into stainless steel pallet, in which the filter paper is cut in size according to the patients' treated area and then soaked (see Fig. 4-5).

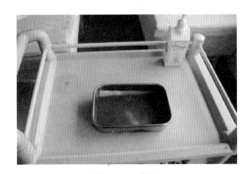

图 4-5　药液

Fig. 4-5　Traditional Chinese medicine liquid

2. 器具准备　电磁炉、煎锅、不锈钢盘、一次性手套、滤纸(尺寸根据患者治疗部位裁取)、热罨包(可调节加热档位)、无菌布。

2. **Appliance preparation**　Electromagnetic oven, frying pan, stainless plate, disposable gloves, filter paper(the size can be cut according to the patient's treated area), hot package(with adjustable heating gears) and bacteria-free cloth.

3. 患者准备　根据穴位依次选取相应的体位进行治疗。

3. **Preparation for patient**　The corresponding body positions of the patient are selected in proper sequence according to acupoints.

4. 皮肤评估　包括色泽、弹性,有无水肿、出血、蜘蛛痣、肝掌、异常隆起、包块及皮下脂肪层厚度等方面指标。

4. **Skin assessment**　Including such indicators as the color, elasticity, whether there are conditions of edema, bleeding, spider nevus, liver palm, anomalous prominence, mass and fat lining thickness.

(二) 操作过程

(Ⅱ) Operation Process

1. 根据穴位嘱患者依次选取相应的体位进行治疗,如仰卧位、侧卧位、俯卧位或坐位。

1. The patient is asked to take the corresponding body positions for treatment in proper order according to acupoints, such as supine position, lateral position, prone position or sitting position.

2. 将浸湿药液的滤纸平铺于患者患处,并加盖一层无菌布,最后将预热好的热罨包置于患处,根据患者情况进行档位温度设置,不宜过热。

2. Lay the medicated filter paper immersed with medicine liquid on the patients' affected area, and then add layer of bacteria-free cloth, finally place the preheated hot package onto the affected area and set the temperature in accordance with the patients' condition, the temperature should not be too high.

如患者体位导致热罨包固定不稳,可加压沙包或用绷带固定,注意不要太紧,以方便紧急情况的处理。

For instability of hot package caused by patients' body position, the sandbags should be pressurized or fixed with bandages, but be noted that the bag should not be fixed too tight in order to make it convenient for treating emergencies.

每日热敷 1 次,每次 20~30 分钟。

The hot package is applied once a day and 20-30 minutes a time.

(三) 操作后处理

(Ⅲ) Treatment after Operation

首先关掉热罨包电源,取下热罨包和塑料薄膜后,施治者应注意慢慢取下滤纸,以防其与皮肤粘连。

First, turn off the hot package power, then, remove the hot package and plastic film. The operator should remove the filter paper slowly in case that there is an adhesion between it and the skin.

最后用纸巾擦拭治疗部位的药液和汗液,嘱患者待汗止后方可离开。

Finally, the operator uses tissues to wipe off the medicinal liquid and sweat on the treated position, and asked the patient not to leave until the sweat stops.

三、临床应用

Ⅲ. Clinical Application

(一) 适用范围

(Ⅰ) Scope of Application

1. 骨科　颈腰椎间盘突出,膝关节炎,肩周炎,类风湿关节炎,骨性关节炎等。

1. In Orthopaedic　Cervical and lumbar vertebrae disc herniation, gonitis, scapulohumeral periarthritis, rheumatoid arthritis, osteoarthritis, etc.

2. 妇科　附件炎,寒凝血瘀型痛经,慢性盆腔炎,月经病等。

2. In Gynecology　Adnexitis, congealing cold and blood stasis type of dysmenorrhea, chronic pelvic inflammation, emmeniopathy, etc.

3. 生殖泌尿　慢性前列腺炎、老年性前列腺增生等。

3. In Genitourinary diseases　Chronic prostatitis, senile prostatic hyperplasia, etc.

4. 儿科　小儿腹胀,腹痛,胃痛,便秘,泄泻等。

4. In Paediatric diseases　Infantile abdominal distension, abdominal pain, gastralgia, constipation, diarrhea, etc.

（二）处方示例

（Ⅱ）Prescription Examples

1. 颈椎病（混合型）

1. Cervical Spondylosis（Mixed Type）

（1）临床表现：颈痛、颈部发僵，上肢放射性疼痛、握力减退，头晕、眼胀，耳鸣，恶心呕吐、心悸等。

（1）Clinical manifestation：Cervicodynia, neck stiffness, radiative pain in upper limbs, holding power decrease, dizziness, eye distension, tinnitus, nausea and vomiting, palpitation, etc.

（2）配方：白芥子 20g、甘遂 15g、延胡索 15g、大黄 20g、芒硝 20g、伸筋草 10g、透骨草 10g、乳香 10g、没药 10g、红花 20g。

（2）Prescription：White mustard seed（20g）, gansui root（15g）, yanhusuo（15g）, rhubarb root and rhizome（20g）, mirabilite（20g）, common clubmoss herb（10g）, speranskia herb（10g）, frankincense（10g）, myrrh（10g）and safflower（20g）.

（3）取穴：大椎、天柱、阿是穴。

（3）Acupoint selection：Dazhui, Tianzhu and Ashi points.

2. 腰椎间盘突出症（寒凝经脉型）

2. Prolapse of Lumbar Intervertebral Disc（Congealing Cold in Meridian Type）

（1）临床表现：腰痛、局部压痛，弯腰困难，遇寒加重，下肢放射性疼痛，行走不利，舌淡苔白，脉沉弱。

（1）Clinical manifestation：Lumbago, local tenderness and difficulty in bending the waist, aggravated by exposure to cold, radiative pain in lower limbs, walking difficulty, pale tongue with white coating, dccp and thin pulse.

（2）配方：白芥子 20g、甘遂 15g、延胡索 15g、大黄 20g、芒硝 20g、伸筋草 10g、透骨草 10g、干姜 30g。

（2）Prescription：White mustard seed（20g）, gansui root（15g）, yanhusuo（15g）, rhubarb root and rhizome（20g）, mirabilite（20g）, common clubmoss herb

（10g），speranskia herb（10g）and dried ginger（30g）.

（3）取穴：肾俞、命门、腰阳关、大肠俞、阿是穴。

（3）Acupoint selection：Shenshu，Mingmen，Yaoyangguan，Dachangshu and Ashi points.

3. 膝关节骨性关节炎（寒凝血瘀型）
3. Knee Osteoarthritis（Congealing Cold and Blood Stasis Type）

（1）临床表现：膝盖肿胀疼痛，遇寒加重，上下楼梯痛，坐起立行时膝部酸痛不适等。

（1）Clinical manifestation：Pain and swelling in knee aggravated by exposure to cold，pain when walking up and down stairs，soreness and discomfort in knee when standing up and walking，etc.

（2）配方：白芥子 20g、甘遂 15g、延胡索 15g、大黄 20g、芒硝 20g、伸筋草 10g、透骨草 10g、独活 20g、牛膝 20g。

（2）Prescription：White mustard seed（20g），gansui root（15g），yanhusuo （15g），rhubarb root and rhizome（20g），mirabilite（20g），common clubmoss herb （10g），speranskia herb（10g），doubleteeth pubescent angelica root（20g）and twotoothed achyranthes root（20g）.

（3）取穴：犊鼻、血海、梁丘、足三里、阳陵泉、阴陵泉、膝阳关。

（3）Acupoint selection：Dubi，Xuehai，Liangqiu，Zusanli，Yanglingquan， Yinlingquan and Xiyangguan.

4. 痛经（气滞血瘀型）
4. Dysmenorrhea（Qi-Stagnation and Blood Stasis Type）

（1）临床表现：行经前后或月经期出现下腹部疼痛、坠胀，伴有腰酸，随着情绪发作症状更甚，舌质紫暗或有瘀斑，脉弦涩。

（1）Clinical manifestation：Lower abdominal pain，swelling of the lower abdomen and sore waist before and after menstruation or during menstrual period， which symptoms are more severe with mood episodes，dark purple tongue with ecchymosis，and stringy and unsmooth pulse.

（2）配方：延胡索 20g、干姜 30g、牛膝 20g、大黄 20g、红花 20g、川芎 20g。

(2) Prescription: Yanhusuo (20g), dried ginger (30g), twotoothed achyranthes root (20g), rhubarb root and rhizome (20g), safflower (20g) and Sichuan lovage rhizome (20g).

(3) 取穴:关元、气海、肾俞、血海、阿是穴。

(3) Acupoint selection: Guanyuan, Qihai, Shenshu, Xuehai and Ashi points.

5. 癃闭(肝郁气滞型)

5. Retention of Urine (Liver Depression and Qi-Stagnation Type)

(1) 临床表现:尿闭,小便量少,点滴而出,甚则闭塞不通,随情绪发作症状更甚,舌红苔白,脉沉弦。

(1) Clinical manifestation: Anuria, oliguria and dribbing, which symptoms are more severe with mood episodes, red tongue with white coating, and deep and stringy pulse.

(2) 配方:延胡索 30g、橘核 20g、大黄 20g、姜黄 20g、荔枝核 20g、牛膝 20g。

(2) Prescription: Yanhusuo (30g), tangerine seed (20g), rhubarb root and rhizome (20g), turmeric (20g), lychee seed (20g) and twotoothed achyranthes root (20g).

(3) 取穴:水道、归来、中极、肾俞。

(3) Acupoint selection: Shuidao, Guilai, Zhongji and Shenshu.

(三) 禁忌证

(Ⅲ) Contraindications

1. 孕妇禁用,妇女月经期腰骶部忌用。

1. It is prohibited for pregnant woman, and the lumbosacral portion is prohibited for women during menstrual period.

2. 外伤后患处有伤口,皮肤急性传染病,特殊体质,贴敷部位有破损者禁用。

2. It is prohibited for traumatic patients with wounds on affected areas, and also for those with acute skin infectious disease, special constitution and damages in the attached positions.

3. 对药物成分过敏者禁用。

3. It is prohibited for patients who are allergic to the pharmaceutical ingredients.

4. 高热、急性化脓性炎症、厌氧菌感染、恶性肿瘤、结核、心肾功能衰竭、心肌梗死、主动脉瘤、出血性疾病、皮肤病、周围循环障碍、严重水肿部位禁用。

4. It is prohibited for patients with hyperpyrexia, acute suppurative inflammation, anaerobic infections, malignant neoplasm, tuberculosis, heart and renal failure, myocardial infarction, aortic aneurysm, hemorrhagic disorders, skin disease, peripheral circulatory disturbance, or on the severe edema position.

(四) 注意事项

(Ⅳ) Precautions

1. 治疗前注意观察患者皮肤表面是否有红肿、皮损或皮肤疾病。

1. Before treatment, the operator should observe whether there are redness, skin lesion or skin disease on the patients' skin surfaces.

2. 选取治疗部位之后再裁剪滤纸的尺寸，尽量做到使滤纸紧贴皮肤。

2. Cut the size of the filter paper after the treated area is selected and try to make the filter paper attached completely to the skin.

3. 确保滤纸浸满、浸透药液，治疗者应先行触碰浸透过中药的滤纸温度是否安全适宜，再将之放置于患者皮肤表面。

3. Ensure the filter paper is soaked and saturated with CMM liquid. The operator should first touch the soaked filter paper to see whether the temperature is safe and proper and then put it on the patients' skin surfaces.

4. 治疗过程中应密切关注患者的温度感觉，保证能随时调整热罨包的温度。

4. During the treatment, pay close attention to patients' feeling of temperature to ensure the temperature of the hot package can be adjusted at any time.

5. 治疗后的滤纸应废弃。

5. After treatment, the filter paper used should be discarded.

6. 药液保持配制新鲜，防止因溶液变质影响治疗效果。

6. The medicine liquid should be kept fresh in case the solution go bad and thus affect the effect.

（五）可能出现的意外情况和处理方法

（Ⅴ）Possible Accidents and Treatments

1. 烫伤出现较小的水疱(直径小于0.5cm)可待其自行吸收,若水疱较大(直径大于0.5cm)则应用无菌针头吸出水疱中的组织液并涂以烫伤膏以避免感染并促进伤口愈合。

1. Small blisters(less than 0.5 cm in diameter)due to scald can be naturally absorbed,and for the larger blisters(greater than 0.5 cm in diameter),the sterile needles should be used to suction out the tissue fluids,and the ointment for scald is applied to avoid infection and promote wound healing.

同时还应注意防止低温烫伤。

In the meantime,low temperature scald should also be prevented.

2. 治疗过程中出现血压升高、心悸等症状时,应立即停止治疗并嘱其静卧休息,如休息后症状没有缓解应立即对症治疗。

2. If such symptoms as blood pressure elevation and palpitation appear during the treatment,stop the treatment immediately and ask the patients to lie down for a rest. If the symptoms are not alleviated,specific treatment should be performed immediately and accordingly.

参 考 文 献
References

[1] 秦小润,汤莉,唐娟,等.中药热奄包治疗湿热瘀阻型盆腔炎性包块临床观察[J].辽宁中医杂志,2014,41(4):737-738.

[2] 李若和,许兵,吴倩,等.中药热奄包对颈椎病患者的临床康复影响[J].浙江中医杂志,2016,51(1):35-36.

[3] 陈世寅,薛亮,罗勇,等.走罐加中药热奄包治疗腰背肌筋膜炎的疗效观察[J].实用医院临床杂志,2015,12(1):144-146.

[4] 祝玲,温贤秀,谭君梅,等.改良中药热奄包法在寒凝血瘀型原发性痛经患者中的应用研究[J].中国计划生育和妇产科,2016,8(10):52-55.

［5］石岩江,杨宏海.中药热奄包为主治疗腰椎间盘突出症临床观察［J］.辽宁中医药大学
学报,2010,12(8):153-154.

第三节 中药湿热敷疗法
Section 3   Therapy of TCM Hot-wet Compress

一、疗法简介

Ⅰ. Therapy Profile

中药湿热敷疗法是一种采用温热的方式来改善局部经络气血的运行,消除风寒湿邪、气血郁滞、痰湿凝滞等病邪,达到邪去正安目的的治疗方法。

The therapy of TCM hot-wet compress is a treatment method that improves the circulation of local meridians, collaterals, qi and blood and eliminates pathogenic wind-cold-dampness, qi stagnation and blood stasis, phlegm-dampness retention, so as to get the goal that the healthy qi returns normal after pathogens are removed.

《厘正按摩要术·熨法》曰:"每遇病者食积痰滞,结于胃脘,宜辛开苦降以治之。设误服攻下大剂,正气已伤,积滞未去,此时邪实正虚,无论攻下不可,即消导破耗之剂,并不敢施,惟有用熨法外治。"辽宁中医药大学附属医院已开展的中药湿热敷疗法,是将加热好的中药蘸于纱布置于身体的患病部位或身体的某一特定穴位上。

The *Revised synopsis of Massage-Hot Medicated Compress* says: "For the patients suffering from the syndrome of food or phlegm accumulated in the gastral cavity, the method of dispelling pathogenic factors with pungency and descending with bitterness should be used. If excessive purgation is taken by mistake, healthy qi will be damaged and food or phlegm stagnancy is not resolved, leading to deficiency of healthy qi and excess of pathogens. In that case, the prescription of promoting digestion and removing the stasis cannot be given, let along that of purgation and only externally used hot compress can be used." Now, the therapy of TCM hot-wet compress has be conducted by Affiliated Hospital of Liaoning University of Traditional Chinese Medicine. It is to put the gauze soaked with heated CMM on the disease sites or certain special acupoints of the body.

中药湿热敷法使药物通过经络之皮部进入血脉,并利用不同药物的性味作用,由经脉入脏腑,输布全身,直达病所,并通过适宜温度刺激,使局部血管扩张,促进血液循环,增加局部药物的强度,改善周围组织的营养,从而具有抑制炎性渗出、消肿止痛、抑制病灶感染、促进血管新生的功效。

The therapy of TCM hot-wet compress makes medicines enter into blood vessels via skin areas of the meridians and collaterals, and makes the medicines enter into zang-fu organs through meridians, and further go all over the body, so as to directly act on the affected sites depending upon different natures and flavours of the medicines. With appropriately thermal stimulus, the therapy also can dilate local blood vessels, promote blood circulation, increase the strength of topical remedy and improve nutrition of surrounding tissue, thereby controlling inflammatory exudation, reducing swelling and alleviating pain, inhibiting focal infection and promoting regeneration of blood vessels.

在脑血管后遗症、骨关节病、软组织损伤疾病的治疗中有着显著的效果,因其方便包裹、温度变化快,尤其适用于小关节痛症,且经济方便、安全无痛,受到广大患者的一致好评。

It has a remarkable effect in treatment of cerebrovascular sequelae, osteoarthrosis and soft tissue injury, and is particularly applicable for small joint pains because of its convenient encapsulation and rapid temperature change. The therapy is also economical, convenient, safe and painless, so it has received unanimous praise from the patients.

二、操作规范

II. Operation Specification

（一）操作前准备

（Ⅰ）Preparation before Operation

1. **器具准备**　电磁炉,煎锅,不锈钢托盘,中药汤剂,无菌纱布,持物钳。

1. **Preparation for Appliance**　Induction cooker, frying pan, stainless steel pallet, CMM decoction, sterile gauze and holding forceps should be prepared.

2. **操作准备**　以中医基础理论为指导,辨证论治,按照一定的剂量将药物进行煎制,将煎好的药汤倒入不锈钢盘内,用消毒的纱布层蘸取热药汤待用。

2. Preparation for Operation　Guided by basic theory of TCM, the doctor should give treatment based on syndrome differentiation, decoct and product medicines according to a certain dose, pour the decocted medical liquid into stainless steel pallet, in which the sterile gauze is soaked for use.

注意随用随做,保证药物纱布的温度(见图 4-6)。

To ensure the appropriate temperature of the medicated gauze, it should be made just before its use(see Fig. 4-6).

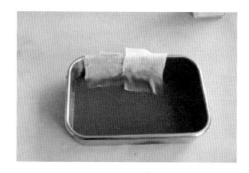

图 4-6　中药液
Fig. 4-6　Traditional Chinese medicine liquid

3. 患者准备

3. Preparation for Patient

(1) 根据穴位依次选取相应的体位进行治疗。

(1) The corresponding body positions of the patient are selected in proper sequence according to acupoints.

(2) 皮肤评估:包括色泽、弹性,有无水肿、出血、蜘蛛痣、肝掌、异常隆起、包块及皮下脂肪层厚度等方面指标。

(2) Skin assessment:Including such indicators as the color, elasticity, whether there are conditions of edema, bleeding, spider nevus, liver palm, anomalous prominence, lump, and fat lining thickness.

(二) 操作过程

(Ⅱ) Operation Process

将煎好的药汤趁热倒入盆内,先取一张消毒纱布蘸取药液,浸湿纱布,轻轻拧干,以平铺打开不滴水为度,放于患处(见图 4-7)。

Pour the decocted medical liquid into a pot, firstly dip a piece of sterile gauze into the liquid, soak the gauze, and gently wring the gauze to the extent that there is no water dripping from it, and put it on affected part (see Fig. 4-7).

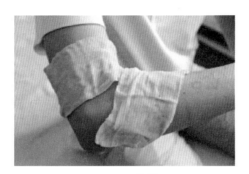

图 4-7　热敷

Fig. 4-7　Hot compress

根据患者的耐受程度，再叠数层，最多可叠到 7~8 层。

According to the tolerance degree of patient, several layers of the gauze, 7-8 at most, can be piled.

如患者自觉温度过高需要更换调整纱布，患者自觉温度减低需将纱布重新蘸取热药汤，再拧干敷于患处。

If the patient feels the temperature is too high, the gauze should be changed, if the patient feels the temperature decreases, the gauze should be once more dipped into hot liquid medicine, wrung out and then put on the affected part.

每日热敷 1 次，每次 15~20 分钟，15~20 日为一疗程。

The hot compress can be used 15-20 minutes once a day, and with a treatment course of 15-20 days.

三、临床应用

Ⅲ. Clinical Application

(一) 适应证

(Ⅰ) Indications

适合于各种闭合性损伤、肢体经络病、关节病、蛇串疮、手指腱鞘炎、足底筋膜炎及网球肘等疾病。尤其适用于其他疗法所不能及的小关节疾病。

The therapy is suitable for various closed injuries, diseases of meridians and collaterals of limbs, arthropathy, snake-like sores, finger tenosynovitis, plantar fasciitis, tennis elbow and other diseases, particularly for facet joint diseases that cannot be cured by other therapies.

（二）处方示例

（Ⅱ）Prescription Sample

1. 蛇串疮（气滞血瘀型）

1. Snake-like Sores（Qi-STAGNANCY and Blood Stasis Type）

（1）临床表现：好发部位依次为肋间神经、颈神经、三叉神经和腰骶神经支配区域。

（1）Clinical Manifestation: Predilection sites are as follows: the regions dominated by intercostal nerve, cervical nerve, trigeminal nerve and lumbosacral nerve.

患处出现水疱，疼痛难忍，沿某一周围神经呈带状排列，多发生在身体的一侧，一般不超过正中线。

The affected part may blister and the pain is unbearable. The blisters are arranged in ribbons along a certain peripheral nerve and always appear on one side of the body, generally not exceeding lineae median.

蛇串疮患者舌质紫暗苔白，脉沉涩。

The symptom of patients with snake-like sores is dark-purple tongue nature, white tongue coating and sunken and astringent pulse.

（2）配方：黄柏 30g、生地榆 30g、五倍子 30g、诃子 30g。

（2）Prescription: Amur cork-tree（30g）, unprepared garden burnet root（30g）, gallnut（30g）and medicine terminalia fruit（30g）.

（3）取穴：局部病变部位。

（3）Acupoint selection: Local diseased region.

2. 肘关节炎（气滞血瘀型）

2. Olenitis（Qi-Stagnation and Blood Stasis Type）

（1）临床表现：非对称性关节痛、关节酸痛，肘关节不能屈曲或者行动受限。

（1）Clinical Manifestation：Asymmetry arthralgia，joint sore，with disturbance of flexion or limitation of movement of elbow joint.

（2）配方：海桐皮 10g、透骨草 10g、路路通 10g、乳香 10g、没药 10g、艾叶 10g、当归 10g、桑寄生 10g、牛膝 10g、独活 10g、川乌 10g、伸筋草 10g。

（2）Prescription：Bark of himalayan coralbean（10g），speranskia herb（10g），beautiful sweetgum fruit（10g），frankincense（10g），myrrh（10g），argy wormwood leaves（10g），Chinese angelica（10g），parasite scurrula（10g），radix achyranthis bidentatae（10g），doubleteeth pubescent angelica root（10g），common monkshood mother root（10g）and common clubmoss herb（10g）.

（3）取穴：局部阿是穴、曲池、少海、小海。

（3）Acupoint Selection：Local Ashi points，Quchi，Shaohai and Xiaohai.

3. 扳机指（瘀血阻络型）

3. Trigger Finger（Static Blood Blocking Collaterals Type）

（1）临床表现：屈、伸指活动过程中，在掌指关节掌侧感觉酸胀、疼痛，比较严重者会出现弹响，甚至绞锁，导致屈、伸指功能障碍。

（1）Clinical Manifestation：The patient feels soreness，distention and pain in palmaris of metacarpophalangeal joints when bending and extending fingers. In severe case，patients may feel a click and even interlocking in metacarpophalangeal joints，resulting in functional disturbance of bending and extending fingers.

晨起时表现较重，午后部分症状有所减轻，寒冷刺激常可加重症状。

Symptoms are more serious in the morning，some symptoms are relieved in the afternoon，and cold stimulation will worsen the symptom.

（2）配方：生大黄 15g、黄连 20g、黄芩 15g、黄柏 15g、红花 20g、没药 20g。

（2）Prescription：Raw rhubarb（15g），golden thread（20g），baical skullcap root （15g），amur cork-tree（15g），safflower（20g）and myrrh（20g）.

（3）取穴：局部疼痛点。

（3）Acupoint Selection：Local pain points.

4. 足底筋膜炎（瘀血阻络型）

4. Plantar Fasciitis（Static Blood Blocking Collaterals Type）

（1）临床表现：脚跟疼痛与不适，压痛点常在足底近足跟处，有时压痛较剧烈，且持续存在。

（1）Clinical Manifestation：The patient feels an ache on his/her heels or has an uncomfortable feeling in the heels, and tenderness points are always on the part near the heels. Sometimes, tenderness is severe and exists persistently.

晨起时疼痛感觉明显，行走过度时疼痛感加剧，严重患者甚至站立休息时也有疼痛感。

The patient feels an evident pain in the heels in the morning, and feels more painful when overwalking. In severe case, the patient may have an painful feeling in the heels even in standing position for a rest.

（2）配方：生大黄 15g、黄连 20g、黄芩 15g、黄柏 15g、红花 20g、没药 20g、牛膝 20g、泽泻 20g、芒硝 10g。

（2）Prescription：Raw rhubarb（15g）, golden thread（20g）, baical skullcap root（15g）, amur cork-tree（15g）, safflower（20g）, myrrh（20g）, twotoothed achyranthes root（20g）, oriental waterplantain rhizome（20g）and mirabilite（10g）.

（3）取穴：局部疼痛点。
（3）Acupoint Selection：Local pain points.

（三）禁忌证
（Ⅲ）Contraindications
1. 外伤后患处有伤口，皮肤急性传染病、特殊体质，贴敷部位有破损者。

1. It is prohibited for the patient who has wound in the affected part, who suffers from acute skin infectious disease, and who has special constitution or whose application position is damaged.

实证、热证、阴虚发热及面部大血管附近慎用。

The therapy should be carefully used for patients with excess syndrome, heat syndrome and fever due to yin deficiency, or to the site nearly facial great vessels.

2. 对药物成分过敏者禁用。
2. It is prohibited for patients who are allergic to the pharmaceutical

ingredients.

3. 高热、急性化脓性炎症、厌氧菌感染、恶性肿瘤、结核、心肾功能衰竭、心肌梗死、主动脉瘤、出血性疾病、皮肤病、周围循环障碍、严重水肿部位禁用。

3. It is prohibited for patients with hyperpyrexia, acute suppurative inflammation, anaerobic infections, malignant neoplasm, tuberculosis, heart and renal failure, myocardial infarction, aortic aneurysm, hemorrhagic disorders, skin disease or peripheral circulatory disturbance or to the site with severe edema.

4. 其他较为严重的内、外科疾病患者禁用。

4. It is prohibited for patients with serious internal and surgical diseases.

(四) 注意事项
(Ⅳ) Precautions

1. 治疗前注意观察患者皮肤表面是否有红肿、皮损或皮肤疾病。

1. Before treatment, the operator should observe whether there are redness, skin lesion or skin disease on the patients' skin surfaces.

2. 药液煮沸后晾 3~5 分钟, 温度以治疗者戴胶皮手套接触温热为度。

2. After it boils, let the medicinal liquid cool for about 3-5 minutes to the point that therapist who wears rubber gloves feels tepid by the hand.

纱布从药液中捞出时, 要拧挤得干湿适度, 以平铺不滴水为度。

When taken out from the medical liquid, the gauze should be appropriately wrung out to the extent that there is no water dripping from the gauze as it spreads out.

3. 纱布的尺寸可根据不同的疾病取穴的需要, 做适当的调整和化裁。

3. The size of gauze may be appropriately changed according to the requirement of acupoints selected for different diseases.

4. 先在患处贴 1~2 层纱布, 观察患者温度感觉并逐渐增加纱布数量, 如已敷满 7~8 层纱布, 但在治疗时间内患者自觉温度下降过快, 应将纱布全部取下并重新贴敷。

4. Put 1-2 layers of gauzes onto the affected part to observe the patient's temperature sensation, gradually increasing the layers of gauzes. If the affected part has been covered with 7-8 layers of gauzes, but the patient feels that the temperature decreases rapidly during treatment, the gauzes should be all removed,

and re-lay the affected part once more.

5. 在应用中药湿敷疗法的同时,还可根据病情适当配合熏洗、药物内服和针灸等疗法,以增强疗效。

5. When applying the therapy of TCM wet compress, the steaming-washing, oral medicine, acupuncture and moxibustion, or other therapies can be used according to the patient's condition so as to enhance the effect.

(五) 可能出现的意外情况和处理方法
(Ⅴ) Possible Accidents and Treatments

1. 治疗过程中观察局部皮肤反应,如出现苍白、红斑、水疱、痒痛或破溃等症状时,立即停止治疗,报告医师,配合处理。

1. Observe local skin reaction during the treatment, if there appear such symptoms as pale, erythema, blister, tickle and pain or ulceration, immediately stop treatment. The operator should report to the physician and cooperatively give appropriate treatment.

2. 烫伤出现较小的水疱可待其自行吸收,若水疱较大则应用无菌针头吸出水疱中的组织液并涂以烫伤膏以避免感染并促进伤口愈合。

2. The smaller blisters due to scald can be naturally absorbed, but for the larger blisters, the sterile needles should be used to suction out the tissue fluids, and the scald ointment should be applied to avoid infection and promote wound healing.

参 考 文 献
References

［1］王会刚,王永静,彭富珍.针灸推拿配合中药湿热敷治疗椎动脉型颈椎病45例临床研究[J].世界中西医结合杂志,2014,9(11):1215-1217.

［2］曾永蕾,孔红兵,王震,等.中药湿热敷配合针刺治疗卒中后肩手综合征30例[J].安徽中医学院学报,2007(4):28-30.

［3］管莉.中药湿热敷配合云克治疗风寒湿痹证型类风湿关节炎缓解关节疼痛的疗效观察[J].全科护理,2015,13(24):2391-2392.

［4］尹梅芳,陈彩,郭丽焕.艾灸配合中药湿热敷治疗带状疱疹后遗神经痛53例疗效观察[J].云南中医中药杂志,2016,37(4):47-48.

第四节　中药蜡疗法
Section 4　Wax Therapy of TCM

一、疗法简介

I. Therapy Profile

中药蜡疗是一种利用加热石蜡和中药封包结合敷在患处,以祛除风寒湿邪的一种传统疗法。

Wax therapy of TCM is a traditional therapy which applies the heated paraffin and CMM bag to the affected part to dispel the cold and dampness.

蜡疗具有恒温性、可塑性、柔韧性等特点,保证了与患处的紧密贴合,石蜡中的化学成分能促进上皮组织生长,同时结合中药的作用,对各类骨病及各种原因引起的软组织损伤效果显著。

The wax therapy has characteristics of homoiothermy, plasticity and flexibility, which guarantees that the wax closely fits to the affected parts. The chemical components of the paraffine can promote growth of the epithelial tissue and simultaneously combine with the actions of the CMM to have notable effect on soft tissue injury caused by various bone diseases and various reasons.

中药蜡疗法首先将无菌纱布封包浸满加热好的中药汤剂,再敷以温热的蜡饼,使之"气闭藏而不泄",局部形成一种汗水难以蒸发扩散的密闭状态,使患处的角质层含水量由 5%~15% 增至 50%,角质层经水合作用,可膨胀成多孔状态,易于药物穿透,不仅能使脂溶性的中药成分穿透皮肤,也能使水溶性成分穿透皮肤,从而使方中的中药充分发挥疗效,取得理想效果。

The wax therapy of TCM is to make the sterile gauze saturated with heated CMM decoction, and then apply the tepid wax cake, to make the gas sealed in the enclosed space without leakage, forming an airtight state, so as to make sweat formed locally difficult to evaporate and diffuse, which makes the water content of stratum corneum in the affected part increase from 5%-15% to 50%. The stratum corneum, after hydration, can be expanded to be poriferous and can make it easy for the medicine to get in, which can not only make the liposoluble CMM components but also the water-soluble components penetrate into the skin, thus making the CMM in the prescriptions exert its therapeutic effect adequately and obtaining an ideal result.

二、操作规范

Ⅱ. Operation Specifications

（一）操作前准备
（Ⅰ）Preparation Before Operation

1. **器械准备**　54号医用石蜡、数码控温智能蜡疗机、电磁炉、煎锅、不锈钢托盘、无菌纱布、弹力绷带、铲刀、棉被。

1. Instrument Preparation　No. 54 medical paraffine, digital control temperature intelligent wax heater, induction cooker, frying pan, stainless steel tray, sterile gauze, elastic bandage, scraper knife and cotton quilt.

2. **患者准备**　根据穴位依次选取相应的体位进行治疗。

2. Preparation for Patient　The corresponding body positions of the patient are selected in proper sequence according to acupoints.

3. **皮肤评估**　包括色泽、弹性，有无水肿、出血、蜘蛛痣、肝掌、异常隆起、包块及皮下脂肪层厚度等方面指标。

3. Skin Assessment　Such indicators as the color, elasticity, presence of edema, bleeding, spider nevus, liver palm, anomalous upheaval, enclosed mass and fat lining thickness should be assessed.

（二）操作步骤
（Ⅱ）Operation Procedures

1. 经过辨证施治后选取适合患者的方药进行煎煮，冷却至45~55℃，将无菌纱布封包浸泡其中15分钟后留置待用。

1. After determination of treatment based on syndrome differentiation, select the prescriptions suitable for the patients to produce the decoction and let it cool to 45-55℃ and immerse the sterile gauze in it for 15 minutes, being ready for use.

2. 蜡箱智能制作蜡饼，其厚度以3~4cm为宜，根据患者治疗部位的选择，将切好的柔软石蜡待用。

2. The wax cake is made in the intelligent wax heater with the thickness of 3-4cm. According to the sizes of treated part selected for the patient, cut the soft paraffine ready for use.

3. 将浸满中药汤液的无菌纱布封包敷于患者患处,尽量全面地接触治疗部位,将蜡饼封包敷于其上,按压使蜡饼形状契合治疗部位,并用弹力绷带捆绑以固定。

3. Lay the gauze, which is saturated with CMM decoction, to the affected parts of the patients, and let it comprehensively contact with the treated part, then lay the wax cake package onto the gauze, press the wax cake to make its shape correspond to the treated part, finally bundle and fix the wax cake package with elastic bandages.

4. 用棉被进行包裹,防止散热过快。

4. Wrap the patients up with cotton quilts to prevent heat loss too fast.

5. 15~20 分钟后取下,废弃封包,将石蜡倒回保温箱进行清洗消毒后备用。

5. Take the packages down after 15-20 minutes, discard the packages and put the paraffine back to an insulation case, and then clean and sterilize it for further use.

6. 治疗时间及疗程:每次治疗时间为 15~20 分钟。

6. Time and course of treatment: The treatment time lasts for 15-20 minutes for one treatment.

风湿骨病类疾病 5~7 日为 1 疗程,神经内科及其他类疾病 10~15 日为 1 疗程。

For rheumatic bone disease, a treatment course lasts for 5-7 days, and for neurological disease and other diseases, a treatment course lasts for 10-15 days.

三、临床应用

Ⅲ. Clinical Application

(一) 适应证

(Ⅰ) Indications

扭挫伤、腰肌劳损、风湿性关节炎、类风湿关节炎、颈肩腰腿疼痛,亦适用于手术愈合、四肢创伤后瘢痕粘连、骨折后肿胀及恢复功能障碍性疾病等。

Sprains and contusions, psoatic strain, rheumatic arthritis, rheumatoid arthritis, pain of neck, shoulder, waist and legs, surgical healing, scar adhesion in limb trauma, swelling in skeletal fracture, recovery period of function disorders, etc.

（二）处方示例

（Ⅱ）Prescription Examples

1. 颈椎病（混合型）

1. Cervical Spondylosis (Mixed Type)

（1）临床表现：颈痛、颈部发僵,上肢放射性疼痛、握力减退,头晕,眼胀,耳鸣,恶心呕吐、心悸等。

（1）Clinical Manifestation: Cervicodynia, neck stiffness, radiative pain in upper limbs, decrease of holding power, dizziness, eye distension, tinnitus, nausea, vomiting, palpitation, etc.

（2）配方：白芥子 20g、甘遂 25g、延胡索 15g、大黄 20g、芒硝 20g、伸筋草 10g、透骨草 10g、乳香 10g、没药 10g、红花 20g。

（2）Prescription: White mustard seed (20g), gansui root (25g), yanhusuo (15g), rhubarb root and rhizome (20g), mirabilite (20g), common clubmoss herb (10g), speranskia herb (10g), frankincense (10g), myrrh (10g) and safflower (20g).

（3）取穴：大椎、大杼、阿是穴。

（3）Acupoint Selection: Dazhui, Dazhu and Ashi points.

2. 腰椎病（瘀血阻络型）

2. Lumbar Spondylosis (Static Blood Blocking Collaterals Type)

（1）临床表现：腰痛、局部压痛,弯腰困难,下肢放射性疼痛,行走不利。

（1）Clinical Manifestation: Lumbago, local tenderness, difficulty in bending waist, radiative pain in lower limbs and disturbance in walking.

（2）配方：白芥子 20g、甘遂 15g、延胡索 20g、大黄 20g、芒硝 20g、伸筋草 20g、透骨草 20g。

（2）Prescription：White mustard seed（20g），gansui root（15g），yanhusuo（20g），rhubarb root and rhizome（20g），mirabilite（20g），common clubmoss herb（20g）and speranskia herb（20g）.

（3）取穴：肾俞、大肠俞、腰阳关、命门、关元俞、阿是穴。

（3）Acupoint Selection：Shenshu，Dachangshu，Yaoyangguan，Mingmen，Guanyuanshu and Ashi points.

3. 类风湿关节炎（寒湿阻络型）

3. Rheumatoid Arthritis（Cold Dampness Blocking Collaterals Type）

（1）临床表现：手、足小关节的多关节、对称性、侵袭性关节炎症，疼痛肿胀，活动不利，有晨僵，病久多伴有关节畸形。

（1）Clinical Manifestation：Symmetrical and erosive joint inflammation，pain，swelling，movement disturbance，morning stiffness and joint deformity of multiple small joints of hands and feet.

（2）配方：羌活20g、威灵仙30g、桂枝20g、川芎20g、细辛20g，白芷15g、姜黄20g、制乳香20g、制没药20g。

（2）Prescription：Incised notopterygium rhizome and root（20g），Chinese clematis root（30g），cassia twig（20g），Sichuan lovage rhizome（20g），manchurian wildginger（20g），dahurian angelica root（15g），turmeric（20g），fried frankincense（20g）and fried myrrh（20g）.

注：可根据治疗需要加入制川乌、制草乌等。

Note：Adix aconiti and radix aconiti kusnezoffii can be added according to needs of treatment.

（3）取穴：阿是穴。

（3）Acupoint Selection：Ashi points.

4. 肩手综合征（瘀血阻络型）

4. Shoulder-Hand Syndrome（Static Blood Blocking Collaterals Type）

（1）临床表现：患手突然浮肿疼痛及肩关节疼痛，并使手功能受限。

（1）Clinical Manifestation：The affected hand suddenly becomes swollen and painful，shoulder joints becomes painful and the hand function is limited.

因疼痛较重并发挛缩。

A heavier pain may be complicated with contracture.

（2）配方：当归 20g、川芎 20g、葛根 20g、红花 20g、白芷 20g、羌活 20g、乳香 30g、没药 30g、伸筋草 20g、透骨草 20g、桑枝 30g、细辛 20g、全蝎 10g。

（2）Prescription：Chinese angelica（20g），Sichuan lovage rhizome（20g），kudzuvine root（20g），safflower（20g），dahurian angelica root（20g），incised notopterygium rhizome and root（20g），frankincense（30g），myrrh（30g），common clubmoss herb（20g），speranskia herb（20g），ramulus mori（30g），manchurian wildginger（20）and scorpion（10g）.

注：可根据治疗需要加入制马钱子等。
Note：Nux vomica can be added according to needs of treatment.

（3）取穴：肩髃、曲池、肩井、外关、阿是穴。
（3）Acupoint selection：Jianyu，Quchi，Jianjing，Waiguan and Ashi points.

5. 肩关节周围炎（瘀血阻络型）

5. Periarthritis of Shoulder（Static Blood Blocking Collaterals Type）

（1）临床表现：肩部逐渐产生疼痛，夜间尤甚，逐渐加重，肩关节活动功能受限而且日益加重，达到某种程度后逐渐缓解，直至最后完全复原为主要表现的肩关节囊及其周围韧带、肌腱和滑囊的慢性特异性炎症。

（1）Clinical Manifestation：Shoulder pain gradually occurs，especially at night and gradually increases，the activity of the shoulder joints is limited functionally and worsen increasingly，and as it gets to a certain extent，the pain will be remitted gradually until it is finally restored. It is a chronic specific inflammation of capsula articularis humeri and its surrounding ligament，tendon and synovial bursa.

（2）配方：防风 30g、红花 20g、威灵仙 20g、川芎 20g、桂枝 20g、桑枝 30g、泽泻 20g、伸筋草 20g、透骨草 20g、延胡索 20g、细辛 20g、生姜 10g。

（2）Prescription：Divaricate saposhnikovia root（30g），safflower（20g），Chinese clematis root（20g），Sichuan lovage rhizome（20g），cassia twig（20g），ramulus mori（30g），oriental waterplantain rhizome（20g），common clubmoss herb（20g），speranskia herb（20g），yanhusuo（20g），manchurian wildginger（20g）and fresh ginger(10g).

（3）取穴：天府、肩髎、肩贞、秉风、肩中俞、肩井、阿是穴。

（3）Acupoint Selection：Tianfu, Jianliao, Jianzhen, Bingfeng, Jianzhongshu, Jianjing and Ashi points.

6. 急性腰扭伤（瘀血阻络型）

6. Acute Lumbar Muscle Sprain(Static Blood Blocking Collaterals Type)

（1）临床表现：急性腰扭伤是腰部肌肉、筋膜、韧带等软组织因外力作用突然受到过度牵拉而引起的急性撕裂伤，常发生于搬抬重物、腰部肌肉强力收缩时。

（1）Clinical Manifestation：Acute lumbar muscle sprain is a kind of acute lacerated wound on parenchyma, such as waist muscle, fascia and ligament, caused by sudden excessive drag with exogenic action. This usually occurs in handling heavy objects or in strong contraction of waist muscles.

（2）配方：当归50g、川芎20g、泽泻30g、牛膝30g、没药30g、三七20g、土鳖虫30g、血竭30g、红花20g，大黄20g、麻黄30g。

（2）Prescription：Chinese angelica(50g), Sichuan lovage rhizome(20g), oriental waterplantain rhizome(30g), twotoothed achyranthes root(30g), myrrh(30g), pseudo-ginseng(20g), ground beetle(30g), draconis resin(30g), safflower(20g), rhubarb root and rhizome(20g) and Chinese ephedrine(30g).

（3）取穴：肾俞、大肠俞、腰阳关、关元俞、秩边、阿是穴。

（3）Acupoint Selection：Shenshu, Dachangshu, Yaoyangguan, Guanyuanshu, Zhibian and Ashi points.

（三）禁忌证

（Ⅲ）Contraindications

1. 对石蜡及药物成分过敏者禁用。

1. It is prohibited for the patients who are allergic to paraffine and drug ingredient.

2. 皮肤感觉障碍、感染及开放伤口处慎用蜡疗。

2. The wax therapy should be cautiously used for the patients with sensory disorder, infection and open wounds.

3. 高热、急性化脓性炎症、厌氧菌感染、妊娠、恶性肿瘤、结核、心肺肾功能衰竭、心肌梗死、主动脉瘤、出血性疾病、皮肤病、严重水肿部位、经深部放射性治疗的患者及 1 岁以下婴儿等禁用。

3. It is prohibited for the patients with hyperpyrexia, acute suppurative inflammation, anaerobic infections, malignant neoplasm, tuberculosis, functional failure of the heart, lung, and kidney, myocardial infarction, aortic aneurysm, hemorrhagic disorders, skin disease, sites with severe oedema, the patients receiving deep radioactive therapy or the infants under one year old.

4. 老年人及儿童在家人陪同下谨慎进行中药蜡疗,经期妇女禁用本疗法。

4. The elderly and children accompanied by family members should be cautiously given the wax therapy of TCM. It is prohibited for the women who are in menstrual period.

（四）注意事项

（Ⅳ）Precautions

1. 石蜡定期清洗、保养、更换。

1. Cleaning, maintenance and replacement are regularly conducted for the paraffine.

2. 经患者创面、溃疡及体腔使用过的石蜡应废弃。

2. The paraffine used on wound surface, ulcer and body cavity of the patients should be discarded.

3. 患者皮肤感觉障碍需要适当降低蜡温,避免烫伤。

3. When the patients have sensory disorder, the temperature of the paraffine needs to be appropriately reduced to avoid scald.

4. 对于开放性伤口,应注意对创面、石蜡及其他材料、用具的消毒,严格无菌操作,尽量选用一次性耗材,治疗后接触创面的材料应废弃,非一次性物品进行严格的无菌消毒,不宜直接反复使用。

4. For the open wounds, a strict sterile operation should be done on the wound surface, paraffine and other materials. Disposable materials are selected as much as possible. The materials contacting with wound surface should be

discarded after use. The non-disposable materials should be sterilized strictly and cannot be directly and repeatedly used.

5. 言语表达不清及运动功能障碍的患者需在家属陪同下治疗。

5. The patients with unclear verbal exposition and dyskinesia need to be treated in the company of the family members.

（五）意外情况及处理方法
（Ⅴ）Treatment for Accidents

1. 出现意外烫伤的患者立即停止治疗，并用冷水冲洗烫伤部位，涂以烫伤膏消炎止痛并促进伤口愈合。

1. For the patients with accidental scalds, the treatment should be stopped at once, and the scalded area is washed with cold water, and the scald ointment is applied to relieve pain and inflammation and promote wound healing.

2. 出现呼吸困难、面色苍白、血压升高的患者停止治疗并采取相应内科疗法诊治。

2. For the patients with dyspnea, pale complexion and elevation of blood pressure, the treatment should be stopped, and the corresponding medical diagnosis and treatment should be adopted.

3. 出现过敏的患者停止治疗。

3. For the patients with allergic reaction, the treatment should be stopped.

参 考 文 献
References

［1］王野,李福生.中药蜡疗结合超短波治疗膝关节滑膜炎疗效观察［J］.中华中医药学刊,
2015,33(8):1876-1879.

［2］王野,白一辰.中药蜡疗结合推拿手法治疗中风后肩手综合征临床观察［J］.中华中医药学刊,2017,35(2):306-309.

［3］黄裕,姚文凤,李哲琳,等.中药蜡疗护理对气滞血瘀型腰椎间盘突出症患者生活质量的影响［J］.中华全科医学,2017,15(1):163-166.

［4］高巧霞.温针灸结合中药蜡疗治疗网球肘的临床观察［J］.光明中医,2017,32(10):
1469-1470.

第五节　中药熏药疗法
Section 5　Fumigation Therapy of TCM

一、疗法简介

I. Therapy Profile

中药熏药疗法是将数味中药研磨成末并混合,然后调制成膏状涂抹于布上,将药布平铺于患者患处,并加以 TDP 神灯在药上进行照射加热。

Fumigation therapy of TCM is a remedy grinding several CMMs into powder and mixed, then preparing the powder into paste and applying it onto cloth, to spread a medicine cloth over the affected part of patient, and to irradiate the medicine by a TDP lamp for heating.

具有温经散寒、行气通络、活血祛瘀、祛风除湿、强筋壮骨的作用。

The remedy has the functions of warming meridians and dispelling cold, activating qi and dredging meridians, promoting blood circulation and removing blood stasis, dispelling wind and eliminating dampness, and strengthening tendons and bones.

优势在于给药途径直接、温和,中药经皮部吸收,安全便捷,同时结合了 TDP 神灯的热效应,使药力更有效地发挥和为机体所吸收。

It has the advantages of direct and mild administration route, safety and convenience because of absorption of CMMs through the skin, at the same time it is combined with thermal effect of the TDP lamp, so that the more medicinal efficacy can exert to the body.

TDP 神灯,由特定加热器(特定的加热温度)加热 TDP 辐射板(用发明专利技术生产的含有 30 多种人体内不可缺少的元素,以无序聚合体、晶态、氧化物和单质元素等物质形态存在,用特殊的制作工艺制成的受专利保护的复合生物搪瓷涂层板),产生波长范围为 2~25μm 的特定电磁波,被与人体细胞中的吸收光谱相吻合的生物体匹配、吸收、传递、转化和利用后产生生物效应,能增强微循环,促进新陈代谢,调整体内微量元素状态、离子浓度、细胞水平和促进生物的信息代谢,加强对人体病变的修复,提高自身的免疫能力。

TDP lamp is used for heating a TDP radiant plate (a composite biological enamel coating plate containing more than 30 indispensable elements in the human body produced using the invention patent technology, existing in form of materials such as unordered polymer, crystalline, oxide and simple-substance element, and made by special production process and protected by patent) by using a specific heater, to generate specific electromagnetic waves within the wavelength range of 2-25μm, which is matched with organisms fitted with the absorption spectra in human cells. So the waves can be absorbed, transmitted, transformed and utilized to produce biological effects, thereby enhancing microcirculation, promoting metabolism, adjusting the state of trace elements, ion concentration and cellular level in the body, promoting information metabolism of organisms, strengthening the restoration of pathological changes of human body, and increasing autoimmunity.

二、操作规范

Ⅱ. Operation Specification

(一) 操作前准备

(Ⅰ) Preparation before Operation

1. 器械准备　中药粉剂、75％酒精、TDP 神灯、无纺布片、不锈钢药缸、压舌板、无菌布、毛巾。

1. Instrument Preparation　CMM powder, 75% alcohol, TDP lamp, nonwoven fabrics, stainless steel medicine mixing can, tongue depressor, sterile cloth and towel.

2. 患者准备　根据穴位依次选取相应的体位进行治疗。

2. Preparation for Patient　The corresponding body positions of the patient are selected in proper sequence according to acupoints.

3. 皮肤评估　包括色泽、弹性, 有无水肿、出血、蜘蛛痣、肝掌、异常隆起、包块及皮下脂肪层厚度等方面指标。

3. Skin assessment　Such indicators as the color, elasticity, whether there are conditions of edema, bleeding, spider nevus, liver palm, anomalous prominence, lump, and fat lining thickness should be assessed.

（二）详细操作步骤

（Ⅱ）Detailed Operation Procedures

1. 将中药打成细粉混合,加入 75% 酒精和水混合成糊状,将调制好的药膏均匀涂抹在无纺布上,厚度 1~2mm,将涂满中药的一面药布向上(药布的大小根据患者治疗部位裁取),未涂中药的一面平铺于患者需要治疗的部位上,再用TDP神灯照射加热,灯头距皮肤的高度 15~20cm(具体根据不同患者对热耐受度调整),20~30 分钟后关闭并挪开神灯灯头,将药布取下结束治疗(如图 4-8)。

1. CMMs are ground into fine powder and then mixed, 75% alcohol and water are added to mix paste. The prepared ointment is uniformly applied to the non-woven fabrics with the thickness of about 1-2mm, with the side of the medicine fabrics fully coated with CMM upwards(the size of the medicine fabrics is tailored according to the treatment part of the patient), the side of the fabrics not coated with CMM is paved on the treated part of the patient, the medicine fabrics is irradiated and heated using a TDP lamp, the lamp cap should be kept away from the skin at a distance of about 15-20cm(specifically, adjusted according to the tolerance level of different patients to heat), the lamp cap is turned off and moved away after 20-30 minutes, the medicine fabrics is taken off, and thus the treatment is completed(as shown in Fig. 4-8).

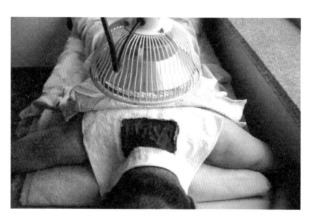

图 4-8　中药熏药疗法

Fig. 4-8　Fumigation therapy of TCM

2. 疗程:每日 20~30 分钟。10~15 天为一疗程。

2. Treatment course: 20-30 minutes every day. 10-15 days makes a treatment course.

三、临床应用

Ⅲ. Clinical Application

（一）适应证

（Ⅰ）Indications

1. **骨科疾病**　退行性骨关节炎、肩周炎、类风湿关节炎、椎间盘突出症、椎管狭窄、椎间关节紊乱等。

1. Orthopaedic Diseases　Degenerative osteoarthrosis, scapulohumeral periarthritis, rheumatoid arthritis, protrusion of the intervertebral disc, spinal stenosis, intervertebral joint disorders and the like.

2. **软伤科疾病**　外伤、劳损所致瘀血性或缺血性关节肌肉疼痛。

2. Soft-tissue Injury Disease　Congestive or ischemic joint and muscular ache caused by trauma and strain.

本项治疗与熥疗的适应证大致相同,药效应强于熥疗,热效应弱于熥疗,二者可以联合治疗。

The indications of this therapy are basically identical to those of Tong therapy, but its medical efficacy is greater than Tong therapy, and its thermal efficacy is weaker than Tong therapy, so that the two can be combined for treatment.

（二）处方示例

（Ⅱ）Prescription Examples

1. **膝关节炎、颈椎病、腰椎间盘突出症**（风寒湿及气滞血瘀型）

1. Gonitis, Cervical Spondylosis and Prolapse of Lumbar Intervertebral Disc (Types of Wind-Cold-Dampness, and Qi-Stagnation and Blood Stasis)

（1）临床表现:患处重着疼痛,肌肉酸楚,关节屈伸不利,得热痛减,舌苔薄白,脉浮弦或沉紧。

（1）Clinical Manifestation: Heavy pain in the affected area, aches and pain of muscles, disturbed flexion and extension of joints, pain relieved by heat, thin white coating of tongue, stringy floating pulse or deep tense pulse.

（2）配方:白芥子20g、甘遂15g、延胡索15g、大黄20g、芒硝20g、伸筋草

10g、透骨草 10g、乳香 10g、没药 10g。

（2）Prescription：White mustard seed（20g），gansui root（15g），yanhusuo
（15g），rhubarb root and rhizome（20g），mirabilite（20g），common clubmoss herb
（10g），speranskia herb（10g），frankincense（10g）and myrrh（10g）.

（3）取穴：内外膝眼穴、血海、梁丘。

（3）Acupoint Selection：Internal and external Xiyan，Xuehai and Liangqiu.

颈椎取穴：大椎、夹脊。

Acupoint selection of cervical vertebra：Dazhui and Jiaji.

腰部取穴：肾俞、委中、腰阳关、命门。

Acupoint selection of waist：Shenshu，Weizhong，Yaoyangguan and
Mingmen.

2. 类风湿关节炎

2. Rheumatoid arthritis

（1）临床表现：手、足小关节的多关节、对称性、侵袭性关节炎症，疼痛肿
胀，活动不利，有晨僵，病久多伴有关节畸形。

（1）Clinical Manifestation：Symmetrical and erosive joint inflammation
of small joints in hands and feet，pain，swelling，disturbed movement，morning
stiffness and joint deformity in prolonged case.

（2）配方：羌活 20g、威灵仙 30g、桂枝 20g、川芎 20g、细辛 20g、白芷 15g、
姜黄 20g、制乳香 20g、制没药 20g。

（2）Prescription：Incised notopterygium rhizome and root（20g），Chinese
clematis root（30g），cassia twig（20g），Sichuan lovage rhizome（20g），manchurian
wildginger（20g），dahurian angelica root（15g），turmeric（20g），fried frankincense
（20g）and fried myrrh（20g）.

（3）取穴：阿是穴。

（3）Acupoint selection：Ashi points.

3. 强直性脊柱炎

3. Ankylosing Spondylitis

（1）临床表现：以脊柱为主要病变部位的慢性病，疼痛，活动不利，累

及骶髂关节,引起脊柱强直和纤维化,造成不同程度眼、肺、肌肉、骨骼的病变。

(1) Clinical Manifestation:A chronic disease with spinal column as the main lesion location,pain,disturbed movement,involvement of sacroiliac joints, causing poker spine and fibrosis,and resulting in different degrees of ocular, pulmonary,muscular and skeletal lesions.

(2) 配方:当归 20g、川芎 20g、木瓜 30g、制乳香 20g、制没药 20g、独活 20g、狗脊 20g、杜仲 30g、伸筋草 30g、川椒 30g。

(2) Prescription:Chinese angelica(20g),Sichuan lovage rhizome(20g), common floweringqince fruit(30g),fried frankincense(20g),fried myrrh(20g), doubleteeth pubescent angelica root(20g),cibot rhizoma(20g),eucommia bark (30g),common clubmoss herb(30g)and Sichuan pepper(30g).

(3) 取穴:督脉、阿是穴、足三里、阳陵泉、三阴交、阴陵泉。

(3) Acupoint Selection:Du meridian,Ashi points,Zusanli,Yanglingquan, Sanyinjiao and Yinlingquan.

4. 泄泻(脾胃虚弱型)
4. Diarrhea(Spleen And Stomach Weakness Type)

(1) 临床表现:大便时泄时溏,食少,食后脘闷不舒,面色萎黄,舌质淡,苔白,脉细弱。

(1) Clinical Manifestation:Diarrhea or semiliquid stool,reduced appetite, stuffy feeling in the epigastrium after meal,sallow complexion,pale tongue with white coating and thready and weak pulse.

(2) 配方:丁香 20g、肉桂 10g、艾叶 20g、雄黄 10g、冰片 5g、干姜 20g、细辛 10g、川椒 10g、白胡椒 10g、吴茱萸 10g、炮姜 20g。

(2) Prescription:Clove(20g),cassia bark(10g),argy wormwood leaves (20g),realgar(10g),borneol(5g),dried ginger(20g),manchurian wildginger (10g),Sichuan pepper(10g),white pepper(10g),medicinal evodia fruit(10g)and baked ginger(20g).

(3) 取穴:神阙、天枢、气海、关元、足三里。

(3) Acupoint Selection:Shenque,Tianshu,Qihai,Guanyuan and Zusanli.

5. 前列腺炎(肾阳不足型)

5. Prostatitis(Insufficiency of Kidney-Yang Type)

(1)临床表现:小腹胀满,时欲小便不得出,或量少无力,面色㿠白,畏寒肢冷,舌淡胖,苔薄白,脉沉细或弱。

(1) Clinical Manifestation:Lower abdominal distension,vesical tenesmus,oliguria or acraturesis,pallid complexion,intolerance to cold with cold limbs,plump pale tongue with white and thin coating and deep thready or weak pulse.

(2)配方:葱白 20g、芒硝 10g、明矾 20g、白胡椒 10g、吴茱萸 15g、大黄 20g、王不留行 15g、花椒 10g、牛膝 15g、冰片 5g。

(2) Prescription:Welsh-onion stalk(20g),mirabilite(10g),alum(20g),white pepper(10g),medicinal evodia fruit(15g),rhubarb root and rhizome(20g),cowherb seed(15g),pricklyash peel(10g),twotoothed achyranthes root(15g)and borneol(5g).

(3)取穴:中极、关元。

(3) Acupoint Selection:Zhongji and Guanyuan.

(三)禁忌证

(Ⅲ) Contraindications

1. 内科疾病　局部皮肤有创伤、溃疡、感染或有严重的皮肤病者。

1. Internal disease　It is prohibited for patients whose local skins have wound,ulcer and infection or for those who have severe diseases.

体质虚弱,高热,结核,恶性肿瘤,出血倾向,重症糖尿病,甲状腺功能亢进,心脏病,高血压,肾功能不全,感染性皮肤病,温热感觉障碍,重症循环衰竭等患者禁用。

It is prohibited for patients who have such conditions as constitutional weakness,hyperpyrexia,malignant tumor,hemorrhagic tendency,severe diabetes,hyperthyroidism,heart disease,hypertension,renal insufficiency,infectious skin diseases,warm sensation disorder and severe circulatory failure.

2. 妇科禁忌　孕妇腹部、腰骶部及某些可促进子宫收缩的穴位,如合谷、三阴交等应禁用,有些药物如麝香等孕妇禁用,以免引起流产。

2. Gynaecological diseases　It is prohibited for pregnant women to be on the abdomen and lumbosacral portion, some acupoints such as Hegu and Sanyinjiao, because the fumigation on these regions or acupoints, and application of such medicines as musk inducing abortion can promote uterine contraction of pregnant women.

经期慎用。

It should be cautiously used for women during menstrual period.

3. **其他**　6 岁以下儿童禁用, 对药物成分过敏患者禁用。

3. **Others**　It is prohibited for children under the age of six and for the patients who are allergic to the medical ingredient.

(四) 注意事项

(Ⅳ) Precautions

1. 检查患者皮肤, 是否有皮损、皮肤过敏或皮肤疾病。

1. The patient should be examined to decide whether there is skin lesion, skin allergy or skin disease.

2. 治疗前检查神灯臂、神灯灯头等部件以免治疗过程中突然滑落发生烫伤。

2. Before treatment, the operator must examine the arm of the lamp, the lamp cap of the lamp and other components to prevent them from sudden falling to cause scalds during the treatment.

3. 根据患者治疗部位裁取布片尺寸, 药膏需要在布片上涂抹均匀, 涂抹厚度在 0.1~0.2cm。

3. Tailor the fabric size according to the treated part of the patient and uniformly daub the ointment on the fabric with the coating thickness of about 0.1-0.2cm.

4. 治疗过程中应密切关注患者的温度感觉, 以防烫伤。

4. During the treatment, the operator should pay close attention to the temperature sense of the patient to avoid scalding.

(五) 不良反应及处理方法

(Ⅴ) Adverse Reactions and Treatment

1. 可能出现的意外情况及处理方法:烫伤出现后较小的水疱可自行吸收,

若水疱较大则应用无菌针头吸出水疱中的组织液,并涂以烫伤膏,避免感染和促进伤口愈合。

1. Possible accident and treatment: The smaller blisters resulting from scalds can be automatically absorbed. However, if the blisters are larger, the sterile needles should be used to suction out the tissue fluids, and the scald ointment should be applied to avoid infection and promote wound healing.

2. 治疗过程中如果出现血压升高、心慌心悸等症状时应立即停止治疗并嘱静卧休息,如休息后症状仍不缓解,则应立即进行对症治疗。

2. If such symptoms as blood pressure elevation and palpitation appear during the treatment, the therapy should be stopped immediately and the operator should ask the patients to lie down for rest. If the symptoms cannot be alleviated through rest, specific treatment should be performed immediately and accordingly.

参 考 文 献
References

［1］张健.TDP神灯中药熏药治疗腰椎间盘突出症的临床疗效观察［D］.沈阳:辽宁中医药大学,2011.

［2］王丽萍.中医理疗治疗强直性脊柱炎的回顾性分析［D］.沈阳:辽宁中医药大学,2016.

［3］孙姗姗.中药熏药配合蜂针治疗类风湿关节炎疗效观察［J］.中医临床研究,2017,9(1):133-134.

［4］宋丽燕.中药熏药治疗痹证的护理［J］.长春中医药大学学报,2008(5):557.